GET WELL
STAY WELL

Reclaim your health
and get back to living

KATHERINE MASLEN ND

First published 2014

Griffin Press
168 Cross Keys Rd
Salisbury South
South Australia 5106

ISBN: 978-0-9925819-0-9

Cover design: Pipeline Designs
Book design: Book Cover Cafe
Author and cover photos: Jason Malouin

National Library of Australia Cataloguing-in-Publication entry

Title: Get well, stay well : reclaim your health and
            get back to living / Katherine Maslen.

Subjects: Health.
            Nutrition.
            Stress management.
            Detoxification (Health).
            Mind and body.
            Self-care, Health.
            Well-being.

Dewey Number:613

CONTENTS

RECIPE INDEX

GRATITUDE

I'd like to express my heartfelt gratitude to many individuals – without their love and guidance, this book would not have been possible.

Firstly to my husband Max, who is my vital support in bringing my message to the world.

To David, Randa and Di, who each ignited my passion for natural medicine and shaped me as a practitioner.

To Kate, who has always offered her unwavering love and support for my success.

To Angie, who has facilitated a large part of my own healing journey.

And to my many patients over the years, who have taught me that miracles happen every day and have inspired me by their commitment to live a better life.

Thank you.

INTRODUCTION
WHAT DOES GOOD HEALTH MEAN TO YOU?

'Health is the thing that makes you feel now is the best time of the year.'
— FRANKLIN P ADAMS

We all know that being healthy is important, but what does having good health mean to you? In my clinical practice I ask my patients this question every day and the answers are always similar:

- 'I want to have the energy to do what I want';
- 'I want to be able to play with my kids';
- 'My mother/father is really sick and I don't want to end up that way';
- 'I'm tired of being worried about my health'; and
- 'I live a really busy life and need to be healthy to keep up with things'.

The common thread is that all of these people recognise the impact that their health can have on the way they live their lives. In fact, health problems can be a real drag.

So the question is, what are you going to do about it? How are you going to get well and stay well so that your body supports you to live a life you love?

You know, I'm not unlike you. I wasn't born a green smoothie drinking, health promoting naturopath. I know exactly what it's like to have health problems and be puzzled about what to do about them. I grew up in a house where consuming soft drink and sweets was a normal part of daily life. When I left home I became a regular binge drinker, smoker and generally ate very poorly. As a consequence I didn't feel great a lot of the time. So what changed?

For me it was a dear friend of mine – Jenny. Jenny had a disease called Systemic Lupus Erythematosus (SLE), which stopped her from living her life the way that she would have liked. She was on a swathe of medication and had limited mobility. In fact, her lupus dictated the way she lived her life. It meant that she could not work or do anything too strenuous, she couldn't venture far from home and it seemed her medication list would keep growing as each new problem arrived. In the end she was very weak and suffered significant pain. I witnessed her condition worsen until her journey finally ended at the age of fifty-two. After she died, I watched as her family were devastated by their loss and I wished that there could have been a better way.

There is. Every one of us has a choice to treat, prevent and avoid illness but we just don't know it yet. When I began to look into our health system, I realised we live in a society which promotes 'sick care' rather than health care, with very little emphasis on looking at prevention rather than cure. We don't know how to look out for the early signs of illness and if we did, our doctors, well-meaning as they are, are trained to treat disease and not imbalance.

Illness doesn't occur by chance. There are underlying causes of illness that allow sickness to occur. This is not an alternative view. Every day there are more and more studies coming out that are giving us clues to the underlying causes of illness – from stress and diet to toxins and environmental factors. We have hundreds of charities which focus on finding a cure, but what if we could simply prevent disease from occurring in the first place? If we could focus on educating people on how to keep healthy and avoid illness, then we'd save billions of dollars in government funding towards 'sick care', improve the genetics of future generations, and have a population whose bodies empower them to live the lives they want, rather than holding them back.

After Jenny's death, I wanted to explore other options of healthcare and my research led me to study herbal medicine and naturopathy. I was so blown away that there was a whole world of effective medicine out there that people didn't know about, that I made it my mission to learn all I could and share it with the world. I have written this book to teach you the basics of preventative health care and to show you that you don't have to wait for disease to occur and take medications to suppress it – there is a better way.

These days I help people overcome their health complaints in my practice every day. It is the most rewarding and fulfilling thing to be able to help patients reclaim their health and feel great. I have helped patients across most conditions – from minor bloating or sleep disturbance, to treating severe period pain, chronic infection and autoimmune disease. There are very few conditions that I have not treated. No matter what the condition though, there is a common framework that I use to make sure that my clients are well.

Over the years I have found that there are seven things that you need to get well and stay well. These are not specific potions or foods or wonder drugs. They are basic concepts that give our bodies what they need to function well so that you can have optimum health.

I have written this book to help you get well and stay well using the same framework that I use with my patients every day. In this book you'll find the basics of what you need to do in your everyday life to achieve wellness and keep your body healthy so you can do the things that you love.

This book is sectioned into three parts that will help you decipher what's out of balance in your body. It will teach you how to get well and stay well. This is how it works:

- The first part is the *diagnosis* – it's about knowing your body and when something goes wrong. If you read the early-warning signs and act on them, you'll be able to avoid illness. In this section you'll learn what 'normal' actually looks like and some great tips and tricks to identify early health issues before they worsen.

- The second part is *education* – now you know what's wrong in your body, what is actually causing these problems? This includes the modern diet, the stress of your lifestyle (did you know that stress causes more disease than smoking and alcohol combined?), And the toxins in your environment (you'll be amazed at the number of things you're exposed to on a daily basis that can harm your health).
- The third part is *taking action* – the steps you can take to reduce or avoid what's triggering your symptoms so you can get well and stay well. These include:
  - **Your diet and nutrition** – I provide an easy-to-follow road map of what will nourish your body without any complicated information about percentages, calories or the like.
  - **Detoxification for health** – You will learn how to support your body's natural detoxification processes with simple seven, fourteen and twenty-one-day detox plans that you can use right now to help your body detoxify.
  - **Relaxation** – Your body needs rest and relaxation so it can get down to the business of healing any symptoms and diseases. Here you'll discover the importance of sleep as well as day-to-day relaxation techniques you can easily incorporate in your life.
  - **Moving your body** – Our bodies are designed to move, and here you will learn how to fit in regular exercise, even if you 'don't have the time'.
  - **Getting outdoors** – You'll find out if you're 'nature deprived' and what that means for your health and wellbeing.
  - **Thinking healthy thoughts** – This is probably the area that gets talked about the least but has the biggest impact, and here you will learn how you can think in a way that boosts your health, rather than weakening it.

I have written this book in a way that you can take any part of it and apply it to your own health. I find that for most people, creating small and manageable changes over time is the best way to truly change your health habits for good, rather than doing an extreme diet or method that only lasts a short period. You'll find easy-to-follow and practical examples of how to apply these methods in your daily life. *Any* improvement in your health that you get as a result of reading this book is a win to me, and of course if you can make several changes across different areas you are well on your way to achieving the health you need to live a life that you love.

To get the most out of this book, I recommend making a checklist of things that you want to change and implementing at least one or two per week. We are a constant work in progress and we learn by repetition – so don't feel disheartened if you try something for a short while and then stop doing it. Come back to your list or re-read sections of this book to reinvigorate yourself and get your health back on track.

I am so excited that you are making some positive changes in your health and I hope that this book helps get you there. The end result will be more energy, less stress, less discomfort and confidence in the fact that you are now aware of what it takes to achieve good health so you can live a life you love.

I believe that good health is essential to living a long and happy life, and I believe that everyone has the right to feel educated and empowered about their health so they can make the right choices. Best of luck with your health journey – I am honoured to be a part of it!

Disclaimer
This book contains advice on how to improve your health using naturopathic principles. It is not meant to give medical advice and should not replace the advice of your doctor. It will, however, provide you with a solid foundation to give your body what it needs to heal. These foundations can be safely used in conjunction with your doctor's advice or other health practitioners' guidance.

PART 1
KNOW YOUR BODY

'The part can never be well unless the whole is well.'
– PLATO

Before you can get well, you need to know what's not working. And, in order to know what's not working, you need to know what it looks like when things *are* working.

One of the issues with the western perspective on health is that most people define 'healthy' as 'not being sick'. I want to change that. I believe there's a big difference between simply not suffering from any illness and truly experiencing health.

So many of us think it's 'normal' to experience regular anxiety, or to have trouble sleeping, or to have low energy, or to have digestive issues. But none of this is normal. When you're truly healthy, your body should support you to do everything you want, rather than holding you back. Your body should easily and regularly eliminate waste. Your moods should be stable and you should sleep deeply. You should have plenty of energy to do everything you want, rather than crashing in the afternoon.

This is healthy. *This* is being well and staying well. And the first step to getting there is to diagnose what *isn't* working, so you can figure out how to fix it.

CHAPTER 1
WHAT'S 'NORMAL'?

*'We have a pharmacy inside us that is absolutely
exquisite. It makes the right medicine, for the precise
time, for the right target organ – with no side effects.'*
– DEEPAK CHOPRA

Although it may seem obvious, the first step to being well is to actually know when things are going wrong. Nearly every condition starts with early-warning signs that tell us that there is a state of imbalance in the body that needs to be fixed.

Our bodies are constantly giving us messages that things are wrong. Signs and symptoms are your body's language – they are there to tell you that there is something wrong on a deeper level so you can take action to fix it. Imagine, for example, that you are about to get a cold. The very first symptoms you might experience are fatigue or achiness – symptoms that you might not even realise were relevant until the more prominent symptoms come about. At this stage the virus has taken hold and you might get a runny nose or sore throat. It is usually here that most people observe that they have caught a cold, often when their immune system is already in full flight trying to fight it. You might then start to look after yourself a little better, maybe taking some vitamin C and rest to get over the illness.

But what if you had done these things right at the very start – before you had an annoying runny nose and that sexy husky voice? If you had listened to the early cues your body was giving you and given your body what it needed (like immune support and rest) it is likely that you wouldn't have been sick for as long or as severely, and potentially not at all.

Paying attention to your body requires you to know what to look for, but also to know what is actually normal. So many of my patients have been told that their symptoms are 'normal' and that they just have to live with them. This is rarely the case and most early signs of illness can be treated easily. So, what exactly is normal?

The truth is that very few people living our modern lifestyles are symptomless 100 per cent of the time. To achieve this most people require low stress and perfect diets, things which ninety-nine per cent of the population lack. But before you know something is abnormal, you first need to know what is normal for your body. Read on to find a breakdown of what normal function looks like, then once you've got a handle on this we'll explore which symptoms are out of the ordinary.

Digestive System

An old naturopathic saying is that all disease begins in the gut. Digestion is an arduous process, requiring more energy than any other process in our bodies. For a perfectly working digestive system, we must have the following:

- A good amount of stomach acid to break down minerals and protein, and to kill pathogens;
- High levels of pancreatic enzymes to break down protein, fat and carbohydrates;
- Regular peristalsis – the movements along the intestines and colon;
- A healthy intestinal microbiome – good levels of health-giving probiotic bacteria and low levels of pathogenic bacteria;
- No insults from allergens or foods which we are intolerant to;
- Adequate water intake; and
- A high intake of soluble and insoluble fibre.

So there is quite a lot that needs to be right for our digestion to do its job properly! Generally speaking, if your digestion is healthy you should notice the following:

- Two to three bowel movements per day, all formed and dark brown in colour;
- Feeling properly evacuated after passing a bowel movement;
- No diarrhoea, constipation or bloating;
- None to occasional wind – rarely smelly;
- No indigestion, pain or discomfort around digestion;
- No burping or bad breath; and
- A healthy appetite.

Urinary System

Our urinary system has the job of filtering out toxins and keeping our fluid levels regulated. Problems with the urinary system are usually due to causes outside this system like infection or blood sugar problems.

The biggest cause of problems with this system is, of course, not drinking enough water, which leads to dehydration. If your water intake is adequate (say one and a half to two litres per day), this is what you should notice:

- Urinating every two to three hours;
- Urine is mostly clear and not cloudy;
- Able to hold urine in (no incontinence);
- Not waking during the night to urinate (even when you don't drink before bed); and
- No pain or discomfort around urination.

Nervous System

Your nervous system includes your brain, spinal cord and nerves. Your nervous system supplies everything in your body, but in particular is associated with symptoms to do with mood, sleep and mental processing. The endocrine system (see below) is also involved in many processes that the nervous system controls.

If your nervous system is healthy you should notice:

- Stable moods – no depression or anxiety (unless circumstantial);
- No shakes, jitters or restlessness;
- You feel calm and focused;
- No headaches, migraines or nerve-related pain; and
- Sleeping well (see endocrine system).

Most of those should be pretty clear, but what do I mean by sleeping well? Sleep is probably the most important thing for our bodies after water (yes – it comes before food!). It is so important that I have dedicated half a chapter to it (see Chapter 9).

Many people think that they sleep well, but did you know that there are ways to measure if you're having the perfect sleep?

In the perfect sleep you will:

- Fall asleep easily – within five to ten minutes;
- Sleep *all* the way through the night;
- Wake up in the morning feeling refreshed; and
- Remember your dreams when you wake up in the morning.

Endocrine System

Your endocrine system is made up of all of the 'endocrine' glands in your body – glands that secrete hormones into your circulation to keep you healthy. Your endocrine system includes:

- Thyroid gland;
- Adrenal glands;
- Ovaries (in women) and testes (in men);
- Pancreas;
- Pineal and pituitary gland; and
- Hypothalamus.

If your endocrine system is healthy and functioning well, you should:
- Have a regular menstrual cycle (women) with minimal pain, no PMS or hormonal symptoms;
- Have a healthy libido;
- Have no mood problems (see nervous system also);
- Be able to cope with day-to-day stressors well; and
- Have good energy levels.

Immune System

Your beautifully complex immune system defends your body from external pathogens. If your immune system is strong you should:
- Not get sick often (less than twice per year);
- Recover from illness quickly;
- Be free from allergies; and
- Be free from dermatitis, eczema and skin infections.

Respiratory System

Your lungs and airways are needed to deliver life-giving oxygen into your blood stream and link to the cardiovascular system. Healthy lung function is an essential part of health.

If your respiratory system is functioning well, you'll notice:
- The ability to breathe without restriction;
- No shortness of breath; and
- No coughing.

Cardiovascular System

A healthy cardiovascular system is needed to pump blood around the body.

If you have a healthy cardiovascular system, you'll experience:
- No palpitations or heart flutters; and
- Good circulation to your extremities.

Integumentary System (Skin)

Your skin is the largest organ of your body and serves many functions, including releasing toxins through sweat.

If you have healthy skin:

- It will be moist and supple;
- Minor cuts will heal well without scarring; and
- You will experience no itching or irritation.

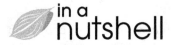

So the gist is that generally we should have great energy, not feel stressed, be sleeping well, not notice our digestion or menstrual cycles too much and have a general sense of wellbeing. Not you? Let's move on then to discover what it means when things go wrong.

CHAPTER 2
WHAT'S WRONG WITH ME?

'The body never lies.'
– MARTHA GRAHAM

Now you know what is normal. And nearly everything that falls outside normal is a signal that your body needs some fine tuning.

A good way to look at it is if you think of your car. You look after it and monitor its health by giving it frequent services to prevent bigger and more costly problems from occurring. You know your car well enough that when it has a small problem with starting or the engine sounds different you get it investigated to find out what's wrong.

Your body needs servicing too. Servicing with good nutrition and rest, but also with the occasional holiday or detox. The poorer your health, the more TLC your body will need. If you listen to your body and service its needs before things get too bad you'll be able to avoid major illness. So what are the signs that things are going wrong?

Signs and symptoms by body system

Digestive signs

There is no system in your body more prone to change than your digestion. Optimum gut function is needed to regulate nutrient absorption, immunity and even moods! The symptoms below are usually signs that there is some dysfunction in the gut – so listen carefully!

Flatulence

Occasional passing of wind is normal due to the fermentation of foods in the colon and intestines. Any wind that is excessive, pain causing or consistently smelly should be seen as a sign of imbalance. This can be from undigested food (low acid or enzymes), bacterial imbalance or inflammation in the gut.

Burping

Burping should not be a regular occurrence under normal circumstances. If you are a 'burper', then usually it means that you have inadequate stomach acid, which leads to fermentation of food in the stomach and release of gasses. If you're burping regularly (and it isn't associated with fizzy drinks) then get it checked out by a naturopath.

Indigestion

Our bodies have an amazingly complex digestive system. If you're getting any form of indigestion, then it means that either part of the system isn't working properly or your body is reacting to something you're eating. Keeping a food diary can help to pinpoint problem foods.

Bloating

Probably the most common symptom that I see in my practice, bloating means that there is maldigestion, irritation or inflammation in the gut. Bloating is when your abdomen – upper or lower (or both) - feels full, puffy or distended. Although the occasional 'full' tummy after an indulgent meal can be normal, any regular and persistent bloating should be investigated by your natural health practitioner.

Bad breath

Bad breath is normally a sign that there is an issue in the stomach. This can be a stomach acid deficiency, which has led to a bacterial overgrowth, or fermentation of food in the stomach. Bad breath can also be caused by saliva that has the wrong pH, bacteria in the mouth and other digestive problems. If you have excess bacteria in the mouth you may need a visit to the dentist.

Pain

Pain anywhere in the body is abnormal – and this goes for your digestion too. Pain means there is cramping or inflammation, or that excess gas is causing stretching of the intestinal or colon wall which leads to pain. Any consistent pain needs to be checked out by your doctor to rule out anything sinister.

Diarrhoea

Having loose bowel movements or diarrhoea means that there is something wrong in the body. It can be due to a food reaction where your body reacts to the food and tries to eliminate it quickly, leading to a decreased transit time and a looser stool. Loose stools can also mean that there is inflammation in the gut or a bacterial, fungal or parasitic issue, particularly if you get diarrhoea every day. Try eliminating dairy and gluten, and if the loose stools persist, it's time for a visit to your health professional. Looser stools can also occur because of stress.

The big two – wheat and dairy

Think you have a food intolerance? It's likely to be dairy or wheat that is the culprit. These are the first foods to eliminate if you are having digestive issues. If this doesn't help, go one step further and take gluten out of the mix too. These foods react most strongly with my patients and often removal of them alone helps to improve symptoms. Try eliminating both for two weeks, then eat a heap of one and see how you feel. Repeat with the other food one week later.

Constipation

Constipation, in naturopathic terms, is anything less than a daily bowel movement. The less frequent, the more severe the constipation is. You are also constipated if your bowel movements are difficult to pass, or you need to strain. Constipation can be something as simple as inadequate water and fibre intake. Like diarrhoea, it can also be due to food intolerance so eliminating the big two – wheat and dairy – can help for some. The health of the microbiome (gut flora) is also really important to prevent constipation. Also consider if stress or tension might be contributing. Try increasing water and fibre intake (fruit, veggies, whole grains, legumes), and avoiding wheat and dairy.

No appetite

Not feeling hungry can be a sign that your stomach acid is low. When our stomach acid is adequate we should feel hungry. A common occurrence is not to feel hungry in the morning, which is often due to particularly low stomach acid after sleeping. Again, stress also needs to be considered. Try having some apple cider vinegar or lemon juice in water before meals to stimulate stomach acid production.

Nervous system and moods

It is normal to have depression and anxiety around significant life events, but it isn't normal to feel the following regularly unless you can pinpoint a reason for them.

Anxiety

When asked if they experience anxiety, a lot of my clients will ask, 'What exactly is anxiety?' Anxiety is one of the symptoms that people often associate with being a normal part of how they feel. Anxiety can range from a feeling of uneasiness in mild cases, to a feeling or worry or dread. Severe anxiety is a feeling that something is going to go wrong, which can even lead to panic attacks for some.

Anxiety can stem from emotional and spiritual causes as well as physical issues like thyroid problems, neurotransmitter imbalances and nutrient deficiencies. Anxiety can also be exacerbated by food intolerances and stress. In any case, if you're anxious or worried without an obvious reason then it is worth getting checked out by a health professional.

Depression

Some of us feel down more than others, but generally if all is well we should feel pretty happy. Depression can arise from a lack of good nutrition, a sleep deficit, neurotransmitter imbalances and hormonal problems. It is also essential to examine if there are emotional causes – even if we're not aware of them.

Is how I'm feeling normal?

Depression and anxiety are both normal occurrences under certain circumstances. It is normal to feel depressed after the death of a loved one or a relationship breakup for a period of time. It is also normal to feel anxiety when you are doing something that is outside your comfort zone, to a certain extent. However, when these feelings happen in your day-to-day activities and without an apparent cause, this is when your body is showing signs of imbalance and might need some help to correct it.

Cranky pants

Are you snappy, short fused or irritable? If it's happening consistently then it could mean that something is up. Common causes are adrenal fatigue, blood sugar regulation issues, hormones or nutrient deficiencies.

Sleep problems

If you're healthy and balanced then you should sleep like a baby. Well, not one of those newborns who keep their parents up all night, but you get the drift. More on this in Chapter 5.

Poor memory or concentration

Where did I put those keys? What time was I supposed to meet my mum? What's his name again? Short-term memory loss is an early sign that your brain is not getting what it needs in the way of nutrition, sleep or stimulation.

Low sex drive

Not feeling enticed by the bedroom anymore? This is often due to excess stress or hormonal problems.

Headaches

Headaches of all types mean that there is something your body is trying to tell you. As a general guide:

- Frontal headaches (forehead) are associated with digestive problems and toxicity.
- Headaches on your temples (temporal) can be due to liver, toxins or muscular tension.
- Headaches behind the eyes are associated with liver issues or sinus congestion.
- Headaches at back or top of the head are usually tension headaches and are due to muscular tension or spinal misalignment (usually both).
- Migraines are more than an early-warning sign and are an indication that there is a severe issue with some element of your health. If you suffer from migraines check in with your doctor first, then look into chiropractic, acupuncture and naturopathy to help.

Endocrine Signs

Because your endocrine glands include the ovaries and testes, some hormonal symptoms are different for men and women.

Hormonal issues

The girls

If you're not on the pill or another form of contraception, your menstrual cycle should be twenty-eight to thirty days, coming at the same time every month. The following period-related symptoms are abnormal and are your body's signs that there is imbalance:

- Pain – any pain that is above 'discomfort' is abnormal and can usually be corrected;
- Large clots in the blood;
- Heavy bleeding or gushing;

- PMS – excessively cranky, irritable, snappy, teary or anxious;
- Fluid retention (you shouldn't get 'fatter' with your period);
- Headaches;
- Breakouts;
- Cravings; or
- Fatigue.

There are very few patients that I have seen that breeze through their periods without any real symptoms. This is because the reproductive system is very delicate and can easily get out of balance. Once you start improving your health you will notice these symptoms begin to reduce and all you should notice is perhaps a mild mood change and the bleeding.

The guys

Any of these fun-to-discuss symptoms can tell you that something is wrong:

- Erectile dysfunction – any problems with getting or maintaining an erection;
- Premature ejaculation;
- Testicular pain or aching; or
- Low libido.

Low testosterone is very common in men and, as well as being one of the causes of the symptoms above, it can also cause fatigue and depression. If you're not feeling great ask your doctor or naturopath to test your testosterone levels. If on the lower end it will cause symptoms. There are many effective herbs to boost testosterone – ask a herbalist or naturopath to find out more.

Thirstiness

Besides not drinking enough water, thirst can mean that you have the beginnings of insulin resistance. If you always need a water bottle on you or drink during the night or wake with a dry mouth then there's a good chance your blood sugar is out of whack. Check in with a naturopath to investigate this further, or your doctor if it is severe.

Floaters in visual field

Floaters, or little specks, in the visual field are normally caused by a lack of blood flow in the eye. The main cause for this is usually high blood sugar levels, which thicken the blood and prevent proper flow.

Excessive sweating

Excessive sweating is usually due to an adrenal response – meaning you have had too much stress. People with adrenal dysfunction often have clammy hands and sweat easily – even without exercise.

Sugar cravings

Sugar cravings are usually a sign of hormonal imbalance and are often the result of poor blood sugar regulation. This, in turn, leads you to eat more sugar and get more blood sugar problems, so it can be a vicious cycle. The more you eat sugar the more you'll crave it. Try avoiding it for a week and notice the change in your body.

Salt cravings

If you regularly crave salty food it can be a sign that your adrenal glands need some TLC, or that your electrolyte balance is out.

 TIP: *An easy thing to do to improve electrolyte balance is to put a pinch of Himalayan or Celtic sea salt in a glass of water every day. This will help give you a wide range of microminerals in addition to sodium.*

Liver Signs

Your liver has a big job, detoxifying almost everything in your body. This includes alcohol, chemicals, heavy metals, excess hormones and fats. If the liver is under prolonged stress, it eventually starts to lose function, which impairs your ability to detoxify, digest and convert hormones in the body.

Nausea

Feeling queasy? If you're not pregnant then it means your liver needs some lovin'. The liver has the job of breaking down any toxins, hormones and metabolites (substances produced through metabolic processes like digestion) so if it's sluggish it can leave you feeling a little ill. Nausea outside pregnancy is not normal and should be checked out by your GP or natural health practitioner.

Alcohol intolerance

Can't handle drinking anymore? This is another sign that your liver needs some TLC. If it can't handle alcohol there's a good chance it's not processing toxins correctly either. See Chapter 8 for help.

Musculoskeletal Signs

Your musculoskeletal system gives you the ability to move, and provides form, support and stability for your body. If this system is out of balance, it leads to symptoms like cramping, pain and discomfort.

Cramping

Muscle cramps are most commonly due to a deficiency of magnesium – from either low levels in the diet or high stress which 'uses up' our magnesium stores. They can also be due to calcium deficiency (less common) and dehydration or electrolyte imbalances.

Body discomfort – musculoskeletal

Discomfort in your body is an early sign that things are wrong. This could be as simple as a postural issue or a lack of the right type of exercise and stretching. If you're active and stretch regularly but still have aches or pains then it is worthwhile seeing a chiropractor, osteopath or musculoskeletal therapist to get to the cause of the issue.

Cardiovascular Signs

If your blood isn't being properly pumped through your body, you might experience the following:

Cold hands and feet

Poor circulation is the most common cause of cold hands and feet. Having good circulation is essential because nutrients get carried around your body through blood flow, and toxins get cleared out as well.

Light-headedness

Light-headedness can be due to low blood pressure, low iron status or low blood volume.

Immune System

Your immune system protects you from external pathogens, so it's not difficult to imagine what could happen if your immune system became imbalanced.

Sneezing

Sneezing is an allergic response from something in your environment, usually dust mites, pollens or animal hair.

Mucous in throat or nose

Your body produces mucous in response to irritation – if it is happening outside of a cold then usually allergy or food intolerance is the culprit. Dairy intolerance will commonly cause a mucousy throat and cutting it out of the diet can help.

Skin and hair signs

Your skin can give you many clues to early dysfunction, and sometimes signs of later disease.

Dry skin

Dry skin is usually due to a deficiency of essential fatty acids (usually omega 3), vitamin E or poor hydration. It can also be a sign that your thyroid is becoming underactive.

Oily skin

Oily skin usually means that your oil producing glands are on overdrive. This can be due to hormones, your thyroid, or sometimes a lack of vitamin A or zinc.

Itchy skin

Your itchy skin is telling you that there is some sort of allergy or irritation going on in the body. It can also mean that your liver isn't breaking down certain compounds, which can make you itchy.

Eczema or dermatitis

Eczema or dermatitis is your body's way of telling you that something is irritating it. This can be food related or an over-reactive immune system may be causing the problem.

Pimples

I could write a whole book on pimples, acne and congestion. For most people, though, a breakout on your face is due to hormones, stress or toxins and if it is congested it could mean you have too many toxins for your body to release – meaning it's detox time (see Chapter 8). Acne is also commonly associated with hidden emotional problems.

Pigmentation

Pigmentation is often a sign that you have too much melanin being produced in the skin. For women it can be due to the hormonal changes associated with pregnancy or the oral contraceptive pill. Improving liver function can help to break down these compounds.

Hair loss

Hair falling out more than it used to? Are your hairs clogging the plug hole? Hair loss can be due to many things but is a sign that your body is in distress. Commonly a deficiency in nutrients (especially iron) has a role, thyroid or hormones can cause it and even stress if it's bad enough. If clumps are coming out then you'll need a visit to your doctor to investigate, then an allied health professional.

Dandruff

Besides using the wrong shampoo, dandruff can be caused by a deficiency of omega 3 and zinc. It can also be caused by food allergies and fungal overgrowth.

Nail signs

Your fingernails can give you a wealth of information about your health. A side benefit of naturopathic treatment is often that clients notice that their nails are stronger and grow faster. This is because of better nutrient levels in the body and improved cellular function.

Nail sign	Meaning
Weak nails	Can be a deficiency in the minerals silica and calcium
White spots on nails	Zinc or calcium deficiency
Pitting (small holes in fingernail surface)	Protein deficiency
Split cuticles	Calcium deficiency
Dry cuticles	Essential fatty acid or vitamin E deficiency
Vertical ridges (lines lengthways)	A deficiency in silica, which is depleted in most Australian soil
Horizontal ridges	In times of extreme stress the nail will stop growing for a period of time – leading to horizontal ridges

Tongue signs

Tongue diagnosis has always fascinated me. I can get so much information from a person just by looking at their tongue for a few seconds. Check your tongue every day and it will give you valuable clues about your health.

A healthy tongue
A healthy tongue should be a pink colour, not pale or red. It should have an even, transparent thin coating and smooth edges. There should be no cracks or lines anywhere.

Tongue sign	Meaning
White coat	'Cold' digestion – lack of enzymes/acid to break down food
Yellow coat	Usually a sign that there is digestive toxicity or congestion
Patchy coating	Can be a fungal overgrowth
Scalloped edges (look serrated)	This is a sign that the liver or gallbladder is dysfunctional
Swollen edges	Digestive dysfunction
Crack down the middle	General digestive weakness – deep seated
Small cracks all over (geographic)	General weakness of connective tissue (the stuff that holds you together). If you have this sign you'll be more prone to varicose veins, sprains and tears, prolapse and the signs of ageing
Bright red tongue	Can be a sign of iron deficiency
Dry tongue	Dehydration
Quivering tongue (shakes when you poke it out)	Magnesium deficiency
Strawberry spots (red dots)	Calcium deficiency

Your symptom status

This list of symptoms is certainly not exhaustive, but you're likely already thinking of things that might be out of the ordinary for you. To delve a little deeper, complete the Health Appraisal Questionnaire from www.katherinemaslen.com/healthcheck to give you further clues as to what might be abnormal for you.

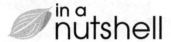in a nutshell

Signs and symptoms are the language your body uses to tell you when something is wrong. By knowing what is abnormal for you, you can act on imbalances early on before they develop into disease. Listen to your body – it is more effective than any blood test.

CHAPTER 3
CATCHING THE EARLY-WARNING SIGNS

*'Modern medicine, for all its advances, knows less than
ten per cent of what your body knows instinctively.'*
– DEEPAK CHOPRA

When you were conceived you were given a unique set of chromosomes from your mother and father that make up who you are. This genetic blueprint holds vital information about you as an individual – what colour eyes you have, your height and even your personality to a certain extent. It also holds your strengths and weaknesses when it comes to your health.

Most of us have at least one health Achilles' heel. And, thanks to our modern lifestyles, our genes are becoming weaker and many of us can have several areas of weakness that we need to look out for.

As well as knowing your genetic history to be more proactive against preventing things like cancer or heart disease, you will have certain health issues that will follow you through your life that will 'play up' in times of high stress or poor nutrition (and you're usually eating crap because you're stressed!).

Take Jane for example. Jane has been seeing me on and off for the good part of a decade to help with digestive problems. Jane knows that each time her diet and lifestyle go off track her digestion is the first place where she experiences symptoms. This is the weak spot of her genetic blueprint.

Knowing your weaknesses gives you the power to prevent the problems they could cause. For Jane, we decided it would be best to put her on a preventative care plan with digestive tonics so that during times of stress, her body would be ready and well-supported for these ups and downs. We also made her keep a diet diary to bring awareness to when she went off track.

My personal Achilles' heel is my skin. From when I was twelve I suffered from acne and it just never seemed to go away. I spent years trying to find answers, taking different supplements, and putting all kinds of things on my skin, from chemical concoctions that bleached my towels to natural skin care. Once I graduated from university and my stress levels dropped I noticed an improvement. It took me years to figure out that when I am stressed it affects my endocrine system and my skin is the first thing to break out. Why? Because that's my weakness. Knowing this now, I am constantly taking preventative measures to make sure I am fully supported nutritionally to deal with stress before it gets out of hand. My skin is such an issue for me that I still get the occasional breakout when things get really hectic, but now I use it as a reminder that I need to slow down and care for my body – it's my early-warning sign that my body needs some TLC.

So can you think of what your weaknesses might be? Perhaps it's your nervous system, which leads to anxiety whenever you are run down. Or perhaps your weak spot is your skin, which breaks out every time your diet goes down the drain. For some people it's their immune system, which leads to frequent colds and flus. Whatever it is for you, pay attention and give this area of your body a little extra TLC. If you're new to this then perhaps checking in with a naturopath to get an overview of your health might help you identify these areas.

Epigenetics and health

Just because you have a weakness it doesn't mean that your body will express it.

Epigenetics is an area that studies the way in which our genes express themselves, and it has shown that you can turn certain genes on and off.

This is determined by factors like diet, lifestyle and toxin exposure, so by eating the right food, looking after your wellbeing and avoiding toxins you can avoid switching on genes that could otherwise cause disease. Very cool indeed!

Self-care plan

Having a self-care plan is an excellent way to make sure that you're putting your health first. Take some time to ask yourself, 'What do my body, mind and spirit need to stay healthy and balanced?'

Some of the things you might like to put on your care plan are:

- Types of foods/meals to include
- Types of foods you need to avoid
- Daily/weekly/monthly rituals that help you keep on top of things – exercise, stretching, baths, reading books, journaling, massage, facials, meditation – anything really!
- Specialist appointments that you need to stay healthy

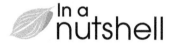 In a

nutshell

We all have a unique genetic blueprint that determines our health, and this includes strengths and weaknesses. By knowing our weaknesses, we can prevent them occurring and act early when things go wrong. Prevention is always better than a cure so remember to look after your whole body and listen to these early-warning signs.

PART 2
WHAT'S THE PROBLEM?

'Your body is a temple, but only if you treat it as one.'
– TERRI GUILLEMETS

Now you know your body. You know what 'normal' looks like, as well as the areas that might be out of balance based on the symptoms you're experiencing. You've also reflected on your weaknesses – the systems that are usually the first to stop functioning optimally when something goes wrong.

So what's causing these problems?

I believe that there are three root causes that have led to the development of disease in our society:

1. The modern diet,
2. Lifestyle stress, and
3. Environmental stress.

It's no secret that the western diet has been on a steady decline over the decades. The poor dietary choices that we make, or are taught to make, have a huge impact on our health – while our bodies will perform as well as they can with the fuel they're given, when this fuel deteriorates, so does our health.

Lifestyle stress comes down to the parts of your lifestyle that trigger stress responses in your body which, over a prolonged period, can lead to disease. Clearly lifestyle stress includes your work, but it also can include elements like your relationships, your daily activities, your diet and even not getting enough sleep.

Environmental stress is triggered by your surrounding environment and, in this day and age, comes down to the toxins we are exposed to in the air, in the products we use and in our food.

Regardless of where the stress comes from, these experiences not only trigger stress hormones in our bodies, but because our bodies are constantly fighting against these diet, environmental and lifestyle factors, they also take away from the resources they could be using to get well.

CHAPTER 4
THE MODERN DIET

'What an extraordinary achievement for a civilisation: to have developed the one diet that reliably makes its people sick!'
– MICHAEL POLLAN

We all know that the food that we put into our bodies determines our health – but are we giving ourselves the right foods? What if many of the foods that you think are healthy, actually *aren't*?

The modern diet is the plague of good health as we know it. We clever humans have managed to use our 'wisdom' to mass produce food, process it so that it lasts for years and make it taste 'delicious' using chemical additives. However, this process had led to a lot of food that is high in calories, but low in actual nutrition.

Before industrial agriculture and intensive animal rearing occurred, before processed foods, before McDonalds and frozen meals, people ate real food. This real food consisted of locally grown fresh fruits and vegetables that were in season, or were naturally preserved for eating later. It consisted of meat raised on open pastures and eggs collected from free-range hens. People consumed milk and cheeses that were made from real milk, straight out of a cow (can you believe it?).

We are far removed from this idyllic scene, where foods were free to roam in their real, wholefood forms. Instead we have perfected the art of mass production and alteration of foods to an extent that has wiped out much of the nutritional benefit and has added a bunch of chemicals along the way. I believe that enough is enough – it is time to reclaim our health by going back to practices that keep the nutrients in our food and respect their unique contribution to our health.

What your dietician isn't telling you

It saddens me to see that dieticians and major health advisers are still promoting some of the most detrimental and nutritionally devoid foods as being good for your health. Unfortunately, we live in a society where the food industry has more sway over the messages we receive than the scientists who have studied food for its health effects. Couple this with the fact that our government doesn't like going back on the things that they have told us, and you have public health messages that tell everyone to eat some of the most detrimental foods out there.

Why does this happen? Like everything, there are usually good intentions at the beginning. Let's look at bread, for example. In Australia, millers are required to add folic acid, a synthetic form of folate, to wheat flour used for bread.

This public health initiative was established to combat the declining rates of folate in our diets, which can increase the risk of neural tube defect in infants. The fact is that folate is naturally present in many grains, including wheat. Yet by processing wheat intensively, the folate in the husk is removed and the remainder destroyed, hence the requirement to add folic acid.

However, this 'solution' misses a core part of the problem, which you discover by asking the question, 'Why were our diets low in folate to begin with?' And the answer is that we simply aren't eating well.

Instead of adding artificial vitamins to nutritionally void food, we need to re-educate people on how to eat nutritional foods. In the bread example, a more useful initiative would be to encourage people to consume bread made from wholegrain flour, which has a far superior nutritional profile and offers much more than just synthetic folate.

So what does this mean for you? Probably, if you haven't figured it out yet, that some of the things you took to be healthy are really not that great for your health after all.

One of the biggest culprits is cereals, which are advertised as being good for you. We also get told that low-fat equals healthy and that dairy is the only real source of calcium. These misleading claims lead many people to try to 'eat healthily', not realising that they are harming their bodies.

Let's examine a typically 'healthy' breakfast of cereal and low-fat milk. It's sold as being high in fibre and low in fat, which must be a good thing, right? It has sultanas – they're healthy aren't they?

On closer examination, though, you'll find that although your cereal is high in fibre, it's nutritionally devoid of much else. Commercial cereals are made by processing and cooking the grains, then shaping them using a process called extrusion. An extrusion machine produces flakes, Os and other shapes using high temperature and pressure. This changes the protein structure of the grains and destroys most of the nutrients they contain. The cereal is then coated in sugar and other flavours to make it taste good.

But what are you really eating? When you look at the label on your cereal box (in fact, the label on any box or packet) it pays to look at the ingredient list, rather than the nutritional panel. We're taught to look for daily percentages and calories, when really this information is confusing and irrelevant if you're eating a healthy, varied diet. Instead, focus on the ingredients.

In the case of a popular Kellogg's cereal, sold to you with images of great health and a slim waistline, the ingredients are:

Cereals (52%) (rice, wheat bran, maize flour, wheat flour),
sugar, whole grains (12%) (whole wheat, wholegrain
oat flour), wheat gluten, oat fibre, minerals (calcium
carbonate, iron, zinc oxide), salt, molasses, flavour, barley
malt extract, rosemary extract, vitamins (vitamin E (soy),
niacin, vitamin B6, riboflavin, thiamin, folate).

Ingredients are listed on a label in order of amounts, with the ingredient that has the highest amount first. At first glance it would appear that this cereal is healthy, with lots of grains and vitamins in it. If you look closely, though, you'll see that sugar comes after the first ingredient cereals (fifty-two per cent), but before whole grains (twelve per cent). This means that the amount of sugar in this cereal could be somewhere between twelve per cent and thirty-six per cent of the total ingredients and, given that the rest of the ingredients are all below twelve per cent, you can expect it to be at the higher end of the range. So your healthy 'wholegrain' cereal actually contains more sugar than it does whole grains.

TIP: *Read the ingredient list, not the front of the box – this will give you clues as to what the product really contains.*

Now, let's look at the milk on your cereal! As far as low-fat milk is concerned, skim milk has been associated with infertility and other health issues (more on this later this chapter), so is not really all it's cracked up to be either.

This commonly eaten breakfast is touted as being healthy, with added vitamins (that's got to be good, right?) and sold to you as being the best start to your day. However, this is not the case, as the label reveals.

What I observe in my practice, is that as soon as people stop eating these toxic foods and replace them with real, wholesome foods, their conditions begin to improve very quickly. Choosing food for its unadulterated nutritional benefits is the only way to get well and stay well.

The uh-uh list: foods you should be avoiding like the plague

Cereal isn't the only bad guy, as far as the modern diet is concerned. In fact, there's a whole list of villains that can throw your body out of balance – I call these the uh-uh list.

These foods are known to cause issues with your health. Now, this doesn't mean that you can never have cake again. But it might mean that you can't have your cake and eat it every day.

There will evidently be times when you eat these foods. That's okay – being healthy is all about moderation. It's about eating amazingly ninety per cent of the time, so that the ten per cent of the time when you do mess up, it doesn't really matter as much. However, these foods should be avoided in your regular diet – that way when you do eat them your body won't suffer in the long term.

Sugar

Sugar, or 'white death' as it is affectionately called by some, is enemy number one in my eyes. It causes more health problems than any other food source.

Now you might think – 'but I don't really have sugar'. Sure, spooning the white death into your coffee is an obvious source, but it is the harder-to-notice sources that add up over the day. You see, sugar is put into foods because we like it. We are hardwired to prefer sweet foods as a higher source of calories.

Back in the caveman days, the more calories we could consume the better. But these days our calorie intake is way more than it should be and sugar is the easiest thing for your body to put straight on to your thighs.

But surely fats make you fat, not sugar? The opposite is actually true – it is very easy for your body to absorb sugar and convert that energy into fat. It is much more difficult for your body to absorb and break down fat to store it as fat.

But what if your weight is not an issue? What if you can eat all of the cupcakes you want without gaining a kilo? Just because we can't see any fat, it doesn't mean it isn't there. The most harmful fat is what surrounds our internal organs. Studies have shown that even those with normal weights can have a high level of fat around the organs. It is this fat that most contributes to your risk of disease.

The other effect of sugar intake is that it causes your pancreas to work harder to break it down. Over time, you can end up with a high-circulating blood sugar, which can then lead to insulin resistance and resulting diabetes. And if you aren't aware of it, diabetes can lead to kidney failure, heart disease, stroke, poor vision, impotence and even the loss of limbs down the track. People with diabetes have a much shorter life expectancy and quality of life due to their illness.

If this wasn't enough to make you turn down that second helping of ice cream, a high intake of sugar also affects the microbiome of the gut, leading to higher levels of candida and fungal overgrowth. Sugar also feeds pathogens and can deplete your immune system.

Blood sugar dysregulation

One of the most common early signs of disease that I see in my practice is blood sugar dysregulation. This happens long before diabetes presents and the signs of high blood sugar are usually quite clear.

Do you get...

- Excessive thirst – especially at night or early in the morning?
- Polyuria – urinating frequently (more than once in two hours with normal water intake of approximately two litres a day)?
- Nocturia – waking during the night to urinate (without a cuppa before bed)?
- Floaters in your visual field (like specks of dust)?
- Sugar cravings?
- Mood swings – especially if you haven't eaten (being 'hangry')?

If you answered yes to two or more of these, then it warrants a visit to your GP or naturopath to check it out.

Sugar isn't always listed on the label as sugar. Look for the following names, which are all different versions of sugar:

- Glucose
- Sucrose
- Fructose
- Dextrose, maltose, lactose (anything ending in 'ose')
- Maltodextrin
- Barley malt
- Brown sugar
- Caramel
- Golden syrup
- Invert sugar

- Cane sugar
- Corn syrup and high fructose corn syrup (these are nastier than conventional sugar and should be avoided)

Foods that probably contain added sugar

- Commercial cereal – Special K, Just Right, Weet-Bix, and more
- Muesli
- Crackers
- Breads
- Dips
- Frozen meals
- Pies
- Store-bought marinades and dressings
- Sauce and condiments
- Premade pasta and stir fry sauces
- Curry pastes
- Canned vegetables
- Canned tuna (flavoured ones)
- Canned and long-life fruit
- Dried fruit – especially cranberries and blueberries

So what is a safe level of sugar to consume? I would be looking at eliminating anything in your everyday diet that contains any sugar whatsoever. If your basic diet is free from added sugars it won't hurt your body so much to have the occasional treat here or there. As a rule, I'd be happy if you ate one thing high in sugar each week or so.

Refined grains

Refined grains are detrimental to our health for several reasons. First, not only are they low in nutrition, but they are 'nutrient robbers' – they take nutrients from your body. This is because in a whole grain, nature has cleverly given us nutrients to process the carbohydrates it contains – chromium, B vitamins and other trace minerals. By taking away the outside of the grain, we remove all of these vital nutrients, leaving just the carbohydrate behind. However, our body still needs to process the carbohydrate, so it takes nutrients from our bodies to do so.

White flour often undergoes a bleaching process as well, making it even more detrimental to your health. Some white flour might even contain traces of aluminium from this process.

Another problem with refined grains is that they spike your blood sugar. Because the fibre is removed they have a higher glycaemic index (GI). Eating large amounts of high-GI food can lead to insulin resistance and diabetes over time, so they are best avoided in your daily diet.

If all of that hasn't got you reaching for your brown rice yet, refined grains also disrupt the digestive system, causing an overgrowth of yeasts and bad bacteria and inhibiting the growth of your friendly bacteria. Next to sugar, refined grains are a large part of the reason why we have so much obesity and illness in today's society.

Glycaemic index (GI) and glycaemic load (GL)

The GI of a food is a measure of what effect it has on your blood sugar – the higher the GI the more your blood sugar will spike when you eat it, and the quicker it will come down. Foods with a lower GI are better for blood sugar regulation as they are released more slowly into the system. A better indicator is the GL, which is more indicative of how the food will be used in the body. Aim for foods with a low GL for maintaining energy levels and preventing diabetes.

Artificial sweeteners

A clue for you – if something has the word artificial in it you probably don't want to be eating it. Artificial sweeteners are just that – pure chemicals that taste like sugar but don't act like sugar in the body... or do they? Although artificial sweeteners don't have any calories, they seem to have a similar effect on the pancreas to sugar.

Aspartame (NutraSweet and Equal)
There are over 900 studies on the detrimental effects of aspartame, and over 10,000 documented reports of adverse reactions, including death. Now while I'm not saying that a can of diet soda will kill you, there are very good reasons not to be ingesting this chemical.

Studies have found that aspartame could cause diabetes just as well as sugar. It increases insulin levels and decreases insulin sensitivity, which are two markers associated with diabetes. Aspartame intake can also cause weight gain (go figure), increase cancer risk and can worsen chronic fatigue syndrome, fibromyalgia, Parkinson's, multiple sclerosis and Alzheimer's. It is a reputed neurotoxin (meaning it can damage your brain and nervous system) and should never be consumed by adults, let alone children.

Sucralose (Splenda)
Sucralose is touted as a biologically inactive compound, but studies would seem to disprove this. Studies on sucralose show that it alters glucose and insulin levels and can metabolise into potentially toxic compounds. Like aspartame, this is best avoided, along with any other artificial sweeteners.

Artificial colours, flavourings and other additives
Although some may be safer than others, generally artificial colours, flavourings and additives are bad news for our bodies.

Would you drink this?

Amyl acetate, amyl butyrate, amyl valerate, anethol, anisyl formate, benzyl acetate, benzyl isobutyrate, butyric acid, cinnamyl isobutyrate, cinnamyl valerate, cognac essential oil, diacetyl, dipropyl ketone, ethyl acetate, ethyl amyl ketone, ethyl butyrate, ethyl cinnamate, ethyl heptanoate, ethyl heptylate, ethyl lactate, ethyl methylphenylglycidate, ethyl nitrate, ethyl propionate, ethyl valerate, heliotropin, hydroxyphenyl-2-butanone (10 per cent solution in alcohol), a-ionone, isobutyl anthranilate, isobutyl butyrate, lemon essential oil, malitol, 4-methylacetophenone, methyl anthranilate, methyl benzoate, methyl cinnamate, methyl heptine carbonate, methyl naphthyl ketone, methyl salicylate, mint essential oil, neroli essential oil, nerolin, neryl isobutyrate, orris butter, phenethyl alcohol, rose, rum ether, g-undecalactone, vanillin and solvent.

These are the chemicals that are needed to make an 'artificial strawberry' flavour. Many of my patients react to artificial colourings and flavourings, reporting symptoms like headaches, anxiety and even allergy symptoms like sneezing.

We don't know what it is that specifically causes problems for people when they consume these additives, but with ingredient lists this big, it's no wonder some people's bodies react.

Artificial colours are also a problem and have been strongly associated with behavioural issues in children and sensitivity in adults.

In Australia there are fourteen artificial colours currently permitted for use, many of which have been banned or restricted in other countries.

Code	Colouring name	Countries which ban or restrict its use	May be found in	Symptoms reported from use
102	Tartrazine	UK, EU, previously banned in Norway	Yellow or orange cordials or sodas, sweets, cake mixes, medicines. Can be combined with 133 to make green foods	Asthma attacks, hives, migraines, blurred vision, itching, over-activity in children
104	Quinoline Yellow	UK, EU, USA, Japan, Canada, previously banned in Norway	Yellow dye found in icy poles, scotch eggs and smoked haddock as well as lipsticks and hair products	Dermatitis
110	Sunset Yellow	UK, EU, previously banned in Norway	Orange squash, orange jelly, marzipan, Swiss rolls, apricot jam, citrus marmalade, sweets, packet soups, cheese sauce, ice cream, canned fish, medications	Hives, rhinitis, nasal congestion, allergies, hyperactivity, kidney tumours, abdominal pain, nausea, vomiting, indigestion

Code	Colouring name	Countries which ban or restrict its use	May be found in	Symptoms reported from use
122	Azorubine, Carmoisine	UK, EU, USA, Canada, Japan, previously banned in Norway	A red dye which is used in marzipan, jams and preserves, sweets, brown sauce, jelly, breadcrumbs, cheesecake mixes	Allergic reactions, rash, fluid retention, hyperactivity
123	Amaranth	USA, previously banned in Norway	Purplish red dye found in ice cream, gravy powder, jams, jelly, tinned fruit, packet cake mix, soups	Allergic/ intolerance reactions, rash, asthma, eczema, hyperactivity
124	Ponceau, Brilliant Scarlet	UK, EU, USA, previously banned in Norway	Desert toppings, jelly, salami, canned strawberries, packet cake mixes, cheesecakes, soups	Allergic/ intolerance reactions, hyperactivity, carcinogen in animals

Code	Colouring name	Countries which ban or restrict its use	May be found in	Symptoms reported from use
127	Erythrosine	Previously banned in Norway	Cherry pink/ red dye found in cocktails, glace and canned cherries, canned fruit, custard mix, sweets, snack foods, biscuits, luncheon meat, salmon spread, scotch eggs, stuffed olives	Phototoxicity, hyperactivity, may interfere with thyroid activity
129	Allura Red	UK, EU, previously banned in Norway	Orange-red colour used in sweets, drinks and condiments, medications, cosmetics	Skin sensitivities, slight allergy/ intolerance reactions
132	Indigotine	Previously banned in Norway	Common in tablets and capsules, ice cream, sweets, baked goods, confectionary, biscuits	Skin sensitivity, rashes, itching, high blood pressure, breathing problems
133	Brilliant Blue	Previously banned in Norway	Processed peas, dairy products, sweets and drinks	Allergy, asthma

Code	Colouring name	Countries which ban or restrict its use	May be found in	Symptoms reported from use
142	Green S	USA, Japan, Canada, previously banned in Norway	Desserts, gravy powder, ice cream, mint sauce, sweets, cake mixes, canned peas	Hyperactivity, asthma, hives, insomnia
143	Fast Green FCF	UK, EU, previously banned in Norway	Sweets, drinks, ice cream, makeup	Bladder tumours in mice
151	Brilliant Black	USA, Canada, Japan, previously banned in Norway	Violet/black dye found in decorations and coatings, deserts, fish paste, flavoured milk drinks, ice cream, red fruit jams, soda, soup and sweets	Allergies, hyperactivity, asthma
155	Brown HT	USA, Canada, Japan, previously banned in Norway	Chocolate flavoured cakes, sweets	Allergies, asthma, skin sensitivity

In 2009 the UK banned what they termed the Southampton Six – six colours that cause significant health concerns – from all food manufacturing. This included sunset yellow FCF (E110), quinoline yellow (E104), carmoisine (E122), allura red (E129), tartrazine (E102), and ponceau 4R (E124). These colours are still used widely in Australia despite the real concern that they pose for our health and the health of our children.

Source: Fed up with food additives – www.fedup.com.au

Preservatives

Preservatives are found in many products like bread, packaged food, wine and smallgoods. The most common preservatives are sulphur preservatives – typically on the label as numbers 220 – 228. Sulphites destroy vitamin B1 – a vital vitamin needed in the body. Many people are sensitive to sulphite preservatives, with reported reactions including anxiety, hives, migraine headaches and asthmatic type symptoms. I recommend avoiding this preservative if you have any allergies, headaches or other sensitivities.

 TIP: *If it's a number, it's not a food – don't consume it!*

Gluten

To gluten or not to gluten, that is the question. Gluten is given a pretty bad rap for good reason – studies have shown that it causes sensitivity in a large portion of the population, and even autoimmune disease (coeliac) in others. Gluten is a protein found in grains like wheat, spelt, rye, khorasan and barley.

Gluten intolerance has developed alongside the increasingly altered state in which we consume these grains. We have gone from eating small amounts of these grains in their whole form, often fermented, to eating massive amounts of super-refined wheat in the form of white bread, pasta, pastries, crackers, biscuits and cakes. Most wheat in Australia is intensively farmed and far removed from the natural organic varieties that our ancestors consumed. There is also the production of 'fast rise' loaves of bread, which use yeast that rises bread in under thirty minutes as opposed to the traditional sourdough method, which could involve rising times of up to twelve hours. This slow fermentation process breaks down the proteins in the grains and unlocks nutrients, making it a much healthier alternative.

Because even a small amount of gluten can cause inflammation in the gut, which is bad news for your digestion and the absorption of nutrients, most people should follow a low-gluten diet, avoiding refined wheat products in particular. While spelt, rye and khorasan also contain gluten, it is in smaller amounts than wheat which makes it easier to digest.

So when shouldn't you eat any gluten?

If you have been diagnosed with coeliac disease – an autoimmune condition which causes your body to react to gluten severely – then you must never eat gluten. This is because not only does your immune system attack the gluten, it also attacks your intestinal wall, leading to damage and eventually maldigestion, which can cause severe nutrient deficiencies.

If you have a family member with coeliac disease, I'd be avoiding gluten too – even if you have been given the all clear there'll be a fair chance that you have sensitivity or the ability to develop sensitivity.

If you get any symptoms from eating gluten – digestive or otherwise – then it is also wise to avoid it as much as possible, or to at least try eating alternative grains like spelt or khorasan.

Gluten has been found to exacerbate irritable bowel syndrome (IBS) and other digestive issues, so if your digestive system is compromised in any way then steer clear of gluten too.

Because gluten affects your immune system, it is wise for those with any autoimmune disease, such as SLE, rheumatoid arthritis, Crohn's disease, ulcerative colitis, psoriasis, Sjorgren's syndrome or sarcoidosis to steer clear of gluten.

Gluten has also been shown to exacerbate those with fibromyalgia, chronic fatigue and asthma.

For people who are healthy without digestive issues or immune problems, a small amount of gluten should not cause too many problems. I would suggest sticking to spelt, khorasan or rye due to their lower gluten content and easier digestibility. If you *are* eating wheat, make sure that it is organic and fermented to ensure easy digestion.

Oats and gluten

Oats are thought to contain gluten but, in fact, they are inherently gluten-free. Oats contain a protein called avenin, which is well tolerated by most coeliac patients.

However, it is recommended that those with coeliac disease avoid oats due to the high level of cross contamination from wheat, rye and barley in the processing plants. Most people can tolerate oats but, if you're very sensitive, make sure you buy oats that are certified gluten-free to avoid this cross contamination.

Low-fat and conventional dairy

Dairy can be problematic for a lot of people. This is due to the way that modern dairy is processed. First of all, dairy is a huge, mass-produced industry – the cows are milked non-stop, even when pregnant, and there are often issues with mastitis so antibiotics are given frequently. The other thing is that the milk that we get today is pasteurised (heated at super high temperatures) and then homogenised (passed through micro-pores to distribute fat evenly).

Pasteurisation is undertaken to kill off any bacteria. Unfortunately, this can also kill off some of the beneficial nutrients that milk contains. Pasteurisation also destroys naturally occurring enzymes that are thought to help with the digestion of the milk proteins.

Homogenisation breaks up the naturally occurring fat globules in milk so that the milk has a uniform, creamy texture rather than the cream floating on top. However, homogenised milk intake has been linked to heart disease and it is thought that it allows the enzyme xanthine oxidase to pass through into the bloodstream, which can damage the arteries and contribute to the build-up of plaque.

Although you can't buy unpasteurised milk in Australia (although you can buy it as 'bath' milk, for 'beauty' purposes), unhomogenised organic milk is becoming easier to buy and I would recommend this for those milk lovers out there.

The other problem with dairy is that low-fat is associated as being healthier, due to the misinformation about saturated fats and heart disease. However, low-fat milk, cheese, yoghurt or other dairy products are a processed food – they are no longer in their wholefood form. This means that your body will not use them the same way that it would if you had the full-fat or whole milk.

One example of where low-fat dairy can be harmful is the case of PCOS (polycystic ovarian syndrome) and infertility. The Nurses' Health Study, which has involved over two-hundred thousand women, found that the more low-fat dairy women consumed, the higher the risk of ovulatory infertility (where you don't ovulate or get a period regularly).

You need to weigh up if dairy is really right for your body – the proteins (casein) and sugars (lactose) in cow's milk are notoriously difficult to digest and many of us simply don't have the capacity to process it. You need to remember that cows' milk is designed by nature for baby cows, with their four stomachs, and not for humans. Symptoms of dairy intolerance are varied and can include diarrhoea, constipation, bowel changes, cramping, indigestion, reflux and mucous in your throat or sinuses.

Dairy can exacerbate some conditions, so avoid dairy if you have any of the following:

- Sinus problems
- Allergies
- Eczema/dermatitis
- Diarrhoea
- Constipation
- Autoimmune disease
- Acne
- Candida/thrush

The lowdown on dairy

Dairy can be consumed as part of a healthy diet, as long as the following criteria are met:

- Must be full-fat
- Must be organic
- Must be unhomogenised
- Must be right for your body type – don't eat if you have any digestive or other symptoms after consumption
- Raw is best, if it is legally available in your country
- Fermented dairy is best – most people tolerate probiotic yoghurts over milk and cheese
- Butter is okay for most as it has negligible lactose and casein present

Trans fatty acids

Trans fats are not naturally occurring fats – they are created as a product of heat or pressure – and are unhealthy because your body cannot use them correctly.

Studies have shown that trans fats are a major contributor to cardiovascular disease and have the ability to increase your 'bad' cholesterol – low density lipoprotein (LDL). People who have high LDL are more prone to heart attacks and strokes. Trans fats have also been shown to stiffen the arteries and increase your risk of diabetes.

Trans fats are found in the following uh-uh foods:

- Margarine and other plant spreads (see pages 112-115 for more info)
- Deep-fried foods
- Potato and other chips made by deep frying
- Shortenings and vegetable oils used in pastry, pies, cakes, biscuits, doughnuts and buns
- Foods cooked with oils that are unstable in heat, like olive oil
- Canned foods with fats in them, due to high temperature canning

The Australian Heart Foundation has recently come under fire for its focus on eliminating saturated fat as a cause of heart disease. The evidence that saturated fat causes heart disease is lacking, but the evidence that trans fats cause heart disease is very strong. The Heart Foundation still recommends margarine over butter and, in fact, margarine products have been given the 'Heart Foundation tick' that indicates that they are heart healthy, even though trans fats are known to affect cholesterol levels. This is a good example of where public health initiatives have gone wrong – giving people the false impression that a food is good for them when, in fact, it is the opposite.

Why I love butter

- It is a stable fat
- It is high in vitamins A, E and D
- It contains butyric acid, which helps heal your gut
- It is low allergen, having very little lactose and casein

Please note that non-organic butter can be a source of toxins – eat organically if possible.

Canned foods

Canned foods are nutritionally depleted and a source of toxins. The process of canning food involves high temperatures over a long period of time to kill off any microbes – this is why canned foods are often very soft and mushy. Any vitamins and minerals that are sensitive to heat are destroyed during this process – especially vitamin C, good fats and many of the B-group vitamins.

Eating canned foods used to run the risk of heavy metal toxicity but these days cans are lined with plastic. This gives you a different toxin – Bisphenol A (BPA), which leaches into your food (more on this in Chapter 6).

Canned food can be a good source of protein and one of the canned foods that you might want to consider is canned fish – particularly salmon that includes the skin and bones or sardines. Although there may be a risk of BPA intake, these foods also contain essential omega 3 fatty acids and calcium so you will need to weigh up the benefit versus the risk in these cases.

Table salt

Table salt, or sodium chloride, is harmful in large amounts because it causes an electrolyte imbalance in the body. This is the salt that is in most canned foods, processed food and ready-made meals.

Salt in itself is not bad; it's just that this type of salt doesn't have any other minerals to support it. Eating sodium chloride on its own can lead to electrolyte imbalances and fluid retention which, in turn, increases blood pressure. Small amounts of Celtic sea salt or Himalayan rock salt are beneficial because they have lots of trace minerals alongside sodium to support health, like iodine, selenium and zinc. These can be included in the diet as meal additives on a daily basis with no risk of harm.

Processed meat

Ham, salami and other cured meats are laden with chemicals and are extremely acid forming (inflammatory) in our bodies.

They are laden with sugar and laced with preservatives that are detrimental to our health.

On top of this, most ham comes from pigs that have been raised in a cage-farming environment which, besides being inhumane, leads to the meat having a poor nutritional profile.

Try to avoid eating ham and deli meats and instead substitute for things like boiled eggs, salmon, sardines (if you can hack them!) and cooked organic chicken meat.

Soft drinks

Drinking soft drinks (soda) is a health hazard that you already know about, but do you know why? Fizzy drinks not only contain loads of sugar or artificial sweeteners, they usually contain a swathe of other chemicals such as artificial colours and flavourings to make them more appealing.

The other thing that you might not know about soft drinks is that they can leach the calcium out of your bones, leading to an increased risk of osteoporosis later in life. This is because they are high in phosphates which, when taken in high amounts, cause high blood phosphate levels. When phosphate levels in the blood are high it reduces the conversion of vitamin D and calcium absorption, which weakens your bones. Phosphorus is highest in cola drinks and soda with sour flavours.

Whole foods versus processed foods

If you haven't realised it yet, I'm a bit of a purist when it comes to food. I like it in its whole, unadulterated form, thank you very much, and you'll notice that many of the uh-uh foods are highly processed. Essentially, the more processing that occurs, the fewer nutrients are left behind so we want to be as close to nature as possible.

Nutrient losses with processing

Nutrient	Cooking losses	Processing losses
Vitamin A	15-35%	Variable
Vitamin B1	40-100%	Milling flour – 60-80% Destroyed by sulphite preservatives
Vitamin B2	10-20%	Variable
Vitamin B3	Heat stable	Ethylene oxide used to ripen fruit – 50%
Vitamin B5	Up to 44%	Milling grains over – 50% Freezing vegetables –50% Canning – 75%
Vitamin B6	30-45%	Milling flour – 75%
Vitamin B12	10-90%	Variable
Vitamin C	Up to 100%	10-90%
Vitamin E	50%	Milling flour – 80%
Essential fatty acids (Omega 3 and 6)	Variable	Hydrogenation destroys a significant amount
Folic acid	65%	Storage loss – 20-75% Milling flour – over 40%
Calcium	Heat stable	Water softeners (used in tap water) remove calcium from drinking water
Iodine	Variable	Refined foods lose most if not all iodine
Iron	Variable	Variable
Magnesium	Variable	Milling wheat – 90%
Selenium	Variable	Milling grains – 40-50%
Zinc	Variable – higher in vegetables	Milling flour – 80% Frozen peas – 25-50% Canning – over 40%

Think about how much of your diet is in its wholefood form, and how much is processed in some way. What percentage of your diet is likely to be nutrient rich, and how much is nutritionally lacking? Now you don't have to be eating whole raw wheat grains, but it would be wise to include whole grains or wholegrain products that are minimally processed, along with fresh fruit and raw or lightly cooked vegetables, raw nuts and seeds and cold-pressed oils, legumes, free-range eggs, wild-caught fish and pasture-raised meats. (We'll dive deeper into this in Chapter 7).

It really is as simple as going back to eating food, rather than food products. We need to get away from eating animals from factory farms and grains that are processed and bleached to what our great grandparents ate. There are very few foods that exist, if any, where intensively processing the food makes it healthier. Change starts with awareness so start thinking about what has happened to your food before it hits your plate.

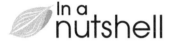

In a nutshell

The modern diet is full of processed, nutritionally devoid food products that are killing us. Additionally, certain foods are worse than others, and are wise to avoid due to the health problems they can create. However, as you learn to see through the crap you will also learn to make healthy choices based on the true benefits of food.

CHAPTER 5
LIFESTYLE STRESS

*'Stress is nothing more than a socially acceptable form
of mental illness.'*
– RICHARD CARLSON

Stress. We all have it to varying degrees, but what does it mean
for your health?

A little stress is actually healthy, but there are very few
people who have 'a little' stress. We are now doing more than
ever, fitting in work, family and everything else in between as we
try to get the most out of life. Now I'm a big believer of living a full
and enriched life, but what if it's slowly killing you?

You might be surprised to know that stress is associated with
more diseases than both smoking and alcohol combined. Stress,
and the accompanying cascade of hormones it creates, can cause
disease and shorten your life span.

So before you say that you're not stressed, as many of my
patients do, let me explain what stress actually is in the body.

Stress is a physiological effect where your body tries to cope
with an upset in the system. Stress can come in many forms
– from the obvious stressors of pressure or being emotionally
upset, to less obvious stressors like a lack of quality sleep, poor
nutrition, pain in the body and having children. When the body
is under stress, your adrenal glands break into action to try and
help you cope.

Your adrenals, and why I keep banging on about them

Your adrenal glands are two small glands that sit right on top of your kidneys. In the event of stress, they pump out a hormone called cortisol, which helps your body deal with the stress.

In the caveman days, this boost of cortisol would help clear your mind and put you into action to get away from a predator or other danger. In those days, our stressors were major. When the fear of being killed by a sabre tooth tiger sets in, your body would go into a sympathetic 'fight or flight' response to help you escape. In this response your body would go into survival mode, diverting all of your energy and blood from the 'non-essential' digestive and reproductive systems to be pumped into your muscles and brain to give you the stamina and mindfulness to get away.

While this response was very useful for getting away from predators, these days we aren't in danger of being eaten. Instead we suffer from low-grade, chronic stressors as a result of our everyday lives. However, because our bodies can't tell the difference between a deadline or a traffic jam and a predator, this still activates our flight or fight response.

What can activate your flight or fight response?

Anything that creates stress activates this response. So, while that can be different for different people, some common examples include:

- **Work issues** – deadlines, issues with your boss, working long hours, a heavy workload, being unhappy at work, being late, and worrying about termination.
- **Family issues** – arguments, fear about a relationship ending, the kids misbehaving, and taking care of sick or elderly family members.
- **Financial issues** – increased financial obligations, losing money, and living pay-cheque to pay-cheque.

- **Significant events** – losing a loved one, losing a job, divorce, getting married and moving houses/cities/countries.
- **Health stress** – pain or discomfort, worry about health complaints, infertility fears, and any uncertainty related to your health.

It's a rare day in the clinic when I don't see any clients that are affected by stress, and it is something I consider for every single patient, regardless of their complaints.

Stress can affect so many aspects of your health and can severely impair the healing process, and I've had so many clients who have struggled to get good results because high levels of stress have sabotaged their treatment.

A good example was Annie, who came to see me for fertility issues. Annie worked in a high stress job as a lawyer doing sixty-hour weeks under an insane amount of pressure. We had been working with Annie for over twelve months, trying to regulate her menstrual cycle and improve her fertility. Although we were able to make some changes, I really felt that Annie's stress was the largest determining factor and that until it was removed she would not fall pregnant. After some discussions, Annie decided to take a few months off to focus on her health. Immediately we noticed that Annie's hormones improved, and one month after she stopped working her PMS was gone, her periods were not as painful and her energy was the best it had been for years. The following cycle she fell pregnant naturally and was over the moon.

As Annie tearfully told me her news it really hit home to me just how much stress can change the course of your life. By removing or reducing external stressors, your body is able to heal and correct itself with ease. Taking Annie out of her constant 'flight or fight' response allowed her treatment to work more quickly and put her into a 'feeding and fornicating' state, which is, of course, more conducive to getting pregnant!

How does stress impact your health?

Regardless of what's triggering your stress response, the ultimate result is that it disrupts the way that your digestive, detoxifying and reproductive organs work. As an example, stress can directly stop your stomach acid pumps from producing acid due to this effect. Stress can also depress the immune system and it interferes with fertility and hormonal health. It literally changes the way your body works.

This is how stress affects your health in the long term:

1. We can end up with high-circulating cortisol levels, which can affect our sleep due to the body's inability to reduce cortisol in the afternoon to initiate the sleep cycle (see Chapter 9 for more info). This is called adrenal overdrive.
2. Over time, the adrenals can get depleted of cortisol, leading to low levels all the time – termed adrenal exhaustion.
3. Once you are adrenally exhausted you can be stuck in a vicious cycle where you can't cope with stress, and the inability to cope causes more stress and more fatigue.

If you think you might be adrenally exhausted, look out for the following:

- Sleep issues – not being able to fall asleep, stay asleep or sleep deeply
- Inability to cope with stress
- Fatigue
- Feeling jumpy, edgy or unable to cope with sudden change

So think about it – are you stressed? Do you have any problems with energy or moods? Do you have any symptoms that may be worrying you or putting stress on your body? Do you worry about things, have anxiety or have a lot on your plate?

Do you have, or are you often around, young children who cause your stress response to go off with every cry or near accident?

Do you work long hours? Do you have problems sleeping? Are you getting less than eight hours of sleep a night? Are you still tired when you wake up?

If you said yes to any of these questions you have some degree of stress.

To get a gauge of how stress is affecting you right now, head over to my website to complete the online Perceived Stress Scale questionnaire at www.katherinemaslen.com/PSS.

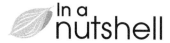 # In a nutshell

---

Stress in the body is one of the major causes of illness. Controlling stress helps your organs to function more effectively and improves your ability to cope on a day-to-day basis.

CHAPTER 6
ENVIRONMENTAL STRESS

'You are a product of your environment. Are the things around you helping you towards success, or are they holding you back?'
– W CLEMENT STONE

Toxins, toxins, toxins. Humans have created them and now humans have to deal with them. They are present everywhere – from the air we breathe to the things we touch to the food we eat.

Put simply, a toxin is anything that has the ability to have a toxic effect in the body, which can damage your cells, your tissues, your organs and, ultimately, your health.

But before we get carried away it's important to note that we are built for detoxifying toxins. Our bodies even create some toxins as a product of metabolism and even healthy foods will contain some compounds that need to be detoxed. We therefore have an amazing capacity to detoxify, as you'll discover in Chapter 8.

The problem is that we are now absorbing small amounts of toxins constantly, which, at a low level or on their own might not pose a health problem, but at a high level and combined with other toxins can have negative effects on your health.

Let's look at the average person's day and what kind of toxins they may encounter:

You wake up in the morning and get into the shower. You wash your hair with your favourite shampoo, which is made up of chemicals like phthalates, parabens and sodium lauryl sulfate (this helps the toxins get into your body more easily). Your body wash contains the same compounds, along with fragrances and colours. If you use a face wash this contains the same compounds.

You step out of the shower, dry yourself and apply your moisturiser (parabens, petroleum oil, fragrance, and formaldehyde). If you're using any hair spray or styling products you can add another hefty dose of phthalates, parabens and other chemicals to the list. If you're applying makeup that day, you can also add more phthalates, parabens, lead and other trace metals. A spray of perfume will really top the list off, being the source of up to 200 chemicals and a concentrated source of phthalates.

You eat breakfast. A healthy breakfast of cereal, milk and berries, which contains pesticide residues that are sources of xenoestrogens. You might also find traces of antibiotics in your milk.

It's time to go to work so you hop into your car. You bought it just a year ago and it still has that new car smell, which is giving off BPA and other chemicals. Sitting in traffic you inhale small amounts of carbon dioxide and petroleum residues which contain formaldehyde and xenoestrogens.

You arrive at work where you get a takeaway coffee, served hot in a paper cup lined with plastic and a plastic top – both of which contain BPA.

For lunch you have some leftovers from home – as well as having pesticide residues it is reheated in a plastic storage container in the microwave, leading to high levels of BPA being leached into your food before you consume it.

You have a can of diet coke with lunch, which is lined with plastic containing BPA, and contains the toxic sweetener aspartame.

Throughout the day you like to keep you water intake up and have a plastic water bottle which you refill from the filter at work. This leaches BPA and probably phthalates into your water.

After work you walk back to your car and on the walk you inhale fumes from cars stuck in traffic during peak hour. These fumes contain xenoestrogens, benzenes and formaldehyde.

Finally at home you sit down to dinner – a bacon quiche that you have with salad. The bacon contains added hormones as well as nitrates and the salad contains traces of pesticides.

After dinner you brush your teeth with a plastic toothbrush with toothpaste, which contains sodium lauryl sulfate and a swathe of other chemicals that are easily absorbed through your mouth.

We are exposed to chemicals every minute of every day. There are multiple studies that show how these toxins affect our health, and this is just the tip of the iceberg when it comes to man-made products and the toxins they contain.

So what are they doing to us?

Pesticides

Many of the toxins we absorb every day are from our food. Pesticides include herbicides (to kill weeds), insecticides (to kill insects), fungicides (to kill fungus) and rodenticides (to kill rodents). Mass farming has led to the use of pesticides to attempt to help with crop yield by poisoning bugs and weeds. I believe that pesticides act like a slow form of poison in our bodies when ingested every day.

There are thousands of chemicals that are used as pesticides, and many of them have been shown to have serious effects on your health. There is mounting evidence that many pesticides act as endocrine disruptors. And, as you know from Chapter 2, when your endocrine system is out of balance this can cause hormonal issues, sugar and salt cravings, excessive sweating, thirstiness and more. Known endocrine disruptors include the chemicals DDT (which is still present in the environment despite being banned for over twenty years), lindazine, atrazine and carbaryl.

Organophosphate pesticides like parathion are used widely in the food chain. They work by irreversibly blocking an enzyme that is essential for brain development in both insects and humans. This is thought to affect the brain development of both foetuses and young children. These pesticides have been linked to an increase in autism spectrum disorders from women who were exposed to pesticides while pregnant and are thought to be harmful to children's brain development, even in low doses. One 2007 study found that the insecticide chlorpyrifos, which is used on some fruit and vegetables, caused a delay in learning rates, reduced physical coordination and was linked to behavioural problems in children, especially attention deficit hyperactivity disorder (ADHD).

Studies have also linked pesticide exposure with non-Hodgkin's lymphoma and leukaemia.

Although there have been many studies on individual pesticides and their health detriments, there have been very few studies that examine the effect of the chemical cocktail of multiple pesticides used together. In the Environmental Working Group's dirty dozen report of the twelve most pesticide-laden fruits and vegetables available in the US, a single grape was found to contain over fifteen different pesticide residues. In my opinion, it is the complex cocktail of chemicals we absorb though our food chain that is one of the underlying drivers of disease. I wholeheartedly recommend organic food to avoid pesticide intake and to help the environment, which, along with your dinner plate, is where many of these chemicals end up.

The dirty dozen and clean fifteen 2014

Every year the Environmental Working Group in the US tests the most widely eaten fruit and vegetables for pesticide residues. The dirty dozen and the clean fifteen are lists of the fruit and veggies that contain the most and least pesticide and herbicide residues. Each year the list changes – visit ewg.org for the latest findings.

The 2014 dirty dozen

Avoid these foods if possible, or buy organic:

1. Apples
2. Strawberries
3. Grapes
4. Celery
5. Peaches
6. Spinach
7. Red capsicum
8. Nectarines
9. Cucumbers
10. Cherry tomatoes
11. Sugar snap peas
12. Potatoes

The 2014 report noted in particular:

- Every nectarine sample and ninety-nine per cent of apple samples tested positive to at least one pesticide residue.
- The average potato had more pesticides than any other food by weight.
- A single grape contained fifteen pesticides.

- Single samples of celery, cherry tomatoes, sugar snap peas and strawberries had thirteen different pesticides in them.

The 2014 clean fifteen

These foods contain few pesticide residues and rarely contain more than one pesticide:

1. Avocado
2. Sweet corn
3. Pineapples
4. Cabbage
5. Peas (frozen)
6. Onions
7. Asparagus
8. Mangoes
9. Papayas
10. Kiwi fruit
11. Eggplant
12. Grapefruit
13. Rockmelon (cantaloupe)
14. Cauliflower
15. Sweet potato

The 2014 report found that:

- Avocados were cleanest – only one per cent of avocado samples had any detectable pesticides.
- Eighty-nine per cent of pineapples, eighty-two per cent of kiwi fruit, eighty per cent of papayas, eighty-eight per cent of mangoes and sixty-one per cent of rockmelons had no residues.
- No single fruit from the clean fifteen tested positive for more than four different pesticides.
- Only 5.5 per cent of the clean fifteen samples had two or more pesticides.

Heavy metals

Heavy metal toxicity has been present for a very long time. The heavy metals arsenic, cadmium, cobalt, lead, mercury and nickel are considered human carcinogens, leaving you at a higher risk of cancer due to their ability to induce oxidative stress in the body. They can interfere with the way that your cells function and can inhibit levels of important minerals, which leads to widespread health effects.

- **Aluminium** – Aluminium toxicity can be found due to its use in products like bleached flour, deodorants and the use of aluminium in vaccines, including the flu vaccine, which some people have annually. Approximately nine per cent of the population have high body levels of aluminium. While aluminium used to be used in cookware, it has largely been replaced by the much safer stainless steel.

- **Mercury** – This is another toxin that is common. It is found in high levels in tuna and other large fish due to its accumulation in the food chain. Mercury is also used as a preservative in some vaccines so young children who can't process the metal well are particularly at risk of mercury toxicity, which can lead to behavioural problems. It has also been associated with autism spectrum disorders.

- **Cadmium** – Cadmium toxicity is common in smokers and passive smokers due to it being in cigarettes. It's also used as a plastic stabiliser in children's toys and many household items. Food that is exposed to glyphosate herbicides like Roundup and other pesticides are also a source of cadmium in the diet.

- **Copper** – An essential nutrient which is needed for health in low levels, but high levels can cause toxicity. In most countries, including Australia and the US, our drinking water comes from copper pipes, which can lead to an accumulation of this mineral. This, in turn, knocks out the competing mineral zinc. I see copper imbalance frequently in people with hormonal issues and infertility. High copper can cause oestrogen dominance and its associated hormonal problems.

* **Lead** – After it was acknowledged that lead caused major health issues like nerve and brain damage and mood disorders, lead use was banned in petrol, paint and other building materials. We now see less severe levels of lead toxicity, but toxicity can still occur, particularly in professionals like painters, mechanics, plumbers and welders who are exposed to high levels. There have been cases of lead toxicity cropping up near areas where lead processing plants were located (always check what was nearby when buying a property). Lead can also be found in cigarette smoke and approximately fifty per cent of inhaled lead can enter the bloodstream.

Heavy metal	Sources	Occupations at risk	Toxicity effects
Aluminium	Aluminium cans Aluminium foil Antacids Anti-diarrhoea medication Antiperspirants Baking powder Bleached flour Cookware Fabric softeners Regional water supplies Toothpaste Vaccines	Aircraft workers Ducting installers Miners Plumbers Refinery workers Welders	Alzheimer's disease Changes in speech or behaviour Exacerbates mercury toxicity Liver dysfunction Loss of bone density Neurotoxicity Parkinson's disease

Heavy metal	Sources	Occupations at risk	Toxicity effects
Arsenic	Pesticides Playgrounds Termite treatments Water Weed killers	Builders Brick layers Bore drillers Carpenters Ceramic workers Concrete workers Gold miners Landscape workers Metallurgists	Cancer (lung, bladder, skin) Confusion Depression Diabetes Hair loss Pigmentation issues Keratosis (scarring) Raynaud's phenomenon
Cadmium	Air pollution Cigarettes Contaminated seafood Household items Pesticides Phosphate fertilisers Toys Water	Carpet layers Jewellers Mechanics Plastics industry Plumbers Toy industry Tyre fitters Welders	Lung cancer Osteomalacia
Copper	Food Water	Electricians Farmers Petroleum industry Plumbers	Fatigue Headaches Insomnia Learning disorders Mood disturbance

Heavy metal	Sources	Occupations at risk	Toxicity effects
Lead	Air pollution Bone meal Cigarettes Ground water Household items Makeup Paints Soil	Fishermen Lead lighting Mechanics Painters Petroleum workers Plumbers Renovators Welders	Abdominal pain Behavioural problems Brain function decline Dizziness Drowsiness Headaches High blood pressure Joint pain Low IQ Mood disturbance Memory loss Tremors
Mercury	Amalgam fillings Body talc Contaminated seafood Fungicides Large fish –shark, swordfish, tilefish, tuna, orange roughy, king mackerel Vaccines	Dental technicians Dentists Gold miners Medical technologists Petroleum workers Sugar cane workers	Asperger's syndrome Autism Autoimmune disease Headaches Hyperactivity Infertility Learning difficulties Nausea Poor memory Sensory loss Tingling of lips and feet Tremor Weakness

Cigarettes (and passive smoking)

You might have noticed that a common item containing heavy metals is cigarettes.

Sadly, if you are smoker I have to tell you that no amount of smoking can be part of a healthy lifestyle. Cigarette smoke contains a swathe of chemicals including cadmium, nicotine, tar, formaldehyde and ammonia. Smoking slows your detoxification, causes fatigue and strips the oxygen out of your cells. And, of course, it can give you cancer too.

Quitting isn't easy and takes a lot. Smoking is a deep habit that can often be masking other emotional issues that haven't been dealt with. So if quitting smoking just isn't possible right now, it would be wise to see a naturopath to get on a supplement regime to correct your nutritional deficiencies and support your body with antioxidants and detoxification herbs.

Passive smoking is another issue which can sometimes be outside of your control. Thankfully, due to smoking laws, smokers can't smoke in many public places now which has helped a lot of people avoid exposure. If you have a family member, partner or friend that smokes, you are still at risk of toxin exposure from cigarette smoke.

You don't have to put up with passive smoking – assert your right to breathe fresh air and kindly ask those around you to refrain from smoking when you're near. Most smokers are kind enough to try and stand away or down-wind of non-smokers so don't be afraid to ask them to move out of your space.

Fluoride toxicity

I'd like to touch on the controversial issue of fluoridating our water supply. Fluoride is found in minute doses in foods like mackerel, sardines, sea salt, sunflower seeds, legumes and tea.

In these minute quantities it has a role in improving bone mass, but not bone strength.

Fluoridated water contains the toxic sodium fluoride, which has no benefit for the body. It is said to prevent cavities by preventing bacterial growth; however, the side effects far outweigh this potential and limited benefit. There have been many dentists who have made an about face when it comes to the promotion of fluoride and a Google search will show you that there is more to this than meets the eye.

Fluoride sits right by iodine in the periodic table, being very similar in biochemical makeup. This means that when you ingest fluoride you are likely displacing iodine in the body, leading to deficiency. Iodine deficiency can cause thyroid problems and increase your risk of breast cancer. Excessive intake of fluoride has been associated with osteosarcoma (bone cancer) and fluorosis of the teeth enamel, which weakens the enamel of your teeth.

Beyond the health ramifications, I believe in having the choice about what goes in to our bodies and mass fluoridation goes against our right to choose what we put into our and our children's bodies.

To remove fluoride from tap water, make sure you filter your water with a filter that removes or reduces the amount of fluoride. You'll also find fluoride in anaesthetics, hypnotic drugs, psychiatric drugs and Prozac.

Chlorine

Like fluoride, chlorine competes with iodine and can also cause deficiency of this important nutrient. It also can harm your microbiome (gut flora). It is therefore imperative to filter chlorine from your water supply to avoid this chemical.

Plastics

Plastic toxins are like the new heavy metals. It took years for lead toxicity to be properly acknowledged and for action to be taken. For plastic toxins, acknowledgement and action is even slower. There are many research papers on toxins found in plastics and their effect in the body, but there has been very little public action on this.

Bisphenol A (BPA)

There are a mounting number of studies that show Bisphenol A's toxicity, but it is still used widely in the production of many plastics that we use every day. BPA has been banned for use in the production of babies' bottles and toys in many countries, including the UK and EU, but is still not illegal in Australia. Many products are beginning to switch to 'BPA-free', but this is a misleading term as, without the use of BPA, other bisphenols are substituted. Commonly Bisphenol S (BPS) is used in BPA-free plastics. BPS has not been studied as extensively as BPA, but preliminary findings are showing that it could indeed be much worse than BPA. Avoiding plastic completely is the only sure-fire way to avoid bisphenol chemicals.

BPA is an endocrine disruptor and xenoestrogen. It has been found to be associated with an increased risk of endometriosis, breast cancer, infertility and even learning difficulties in children. There have also been studies linking it to impotence, diabetes, heart disease and asthma.

Studies by the CDC (centre for disease control) in America found that ninety-five per cent of adults had detectable levels of BPA in their bodies, as did ninety-three per cent of children. As more and more studies come out linking BPA to serious health effects, we need to rethink the way that we use these plastics in our day-to-day lives.

De-plastic your life

Avoiding plastic use is one of the easy ways you can help reduce your intake of BPA and phthalates. As you'll find while trying to reduce use – it's nearly impossible to avoid plastics altogether, but making a few major changes should help to reduce your exposure.

- Use a glass or stainless steel water bottle, preferably filled up from a tap with a water filter attached.
- Avoid putting food in plastic containers – instead use glass storage containers, ceramic or stainless steel.
- Never heat food in plastic containers. Never!
- Get rid of any plastic utensils, cooking equipment, cups, plates or cutlery. Instead use stainless steel utensils or wood for non-stick pans. For kids use wooden or stainless steel plates and cups.
- Avoid the use of plastic wrap – especially directly on food.
- Reduce the intake of canned food and drinks – which are lined with plastic.
- Think about where else you might be exposed to plastics. Could you find an alternative?

Phthalates

Phthalates (pronounced tha-lates) are toxic chemicals found in plastics, personal care products and other commonly used items. They have been linked to a broad range of health detriments, including increases in breast cancer, endometriosis, hormonal problems and infertility.

Phthalates have been found to be a contributing factor to asthma, diabetes, preterm birth and issues like obesity, ADHD and other behavioural problems in children. Studies have shown that intake during pregnancy can lead to defects of the genitals in male babies and low testosterone. One study even found that high phthalate levels during pregnancy was associated with feminisation in young boys, with less male-type behaviour like rough and tumble play.

If you're shocked about what phthalates have the potential to do, you'll be even more astonished to learn that you are touching, using and absorbing phthalates every single day. Phthalates are commonly used in cosmetics and personal care products, including soap, body wash, perfume, hair spray, shampoo, nail polish, cleansers, toners and moisturisers. They're also used as a plasticiser to soften plastic and vinyl toys, shower curtains, wallpaper, food packaging, and plastic wrap. Other sources include wood finishes, detergents, adhesives, plastic plumbing pipes, lubricants, medical tubing and fluid bags (IV of phthalates with your medicine?), solvents, insecticides, building materials, and vinyl flooring. If you see a soft and pliable plastic it will likely be high in phthalates. Phthalates are also in babies' toys and teething rings – these 'phthalate lollipops' have the ability to disrupt our children's endocrine systems from a very young age.

Phthalates are easily absorbed into the human body, and it is no wonder since we come into contact with them thousands of times throughout our lives. More and more studies are coming out linking urinary phthalate levels to health problems. There was a notable study in the Journal of Paediatrics in 2013 linking urinary phthalates to increases in blood pressure in children, and at the time of writing this book there was a paper released online linking urinary phthalates output to lower testosterone levels in men, women and children.

Although phthalates have been proven to cause or contribute to a wide range of diseases, there is no regulation of their use in Australia. You will still find Phthalates in babies' toys, skin care and plastic food storage containers.

Every patient that we have ever screened at our health centre has had detectable levels of phthalates in their urine.

Plastic and the environment

Reducing your plastic use not only is a great move for your health but will help the environment too. Plastics never break down, so every plastic bottle, cup, straw, bag or other plastic item ever created is still on this Earth – much of it in our oceans killing birds and sea life. By consciously reducing your use of plastic you can help to reduce the environmental impact of this detrimental substance.

Toxins in personal care products

Unlike food products, there is no regulation for the things that go in to skin care, even though it is well known that you can absorb chemicals through the skin. We know from studies that show urinary elimination of skincare chemicals that we absorb a significant percentage of what is put on our skin.

Many products that are put in personal care products like body wash, shampoo, conditioner, moisturisers, styling products and makeup are very toxic and have the research to prove it. As well as phthalates, which we've already covered in detail, the following chemicals have been shown to harm your health.

Parabens

Listed as methylparabens, propylparaben, butylparaben or ethylparaben; parabens are hormone disruptors. This means that they can get into your body and create hormonal imbalances due to their xenoestrogenic effect. Parabens have been found in breast cancer tissue and have been found to interfere with male hormonal function.

One study found that methylparaben used on the skin reacts with UVB rays, leading to increased skin aging and DNA damage.

This is bad news if you're trying to avoid skin cancer (and yes, parabens are in sunscreens).

It stresses me to see that parabens are one of the main ingredients in baby products – baby wipes, which are used up to six times a day on infants until they are at least eighteen months old, are a direct source of parabens into their bodies through the fragile skin in the genital area. If you look at some makeup and moisturisers, you'll see that methylparaben is the main component that is 'nourishing' your skin.

Synthetic parabens should be banned in any product that is destined to stay on your body. In fact, they should be banned for good. This is one area of toxins we can easily avoid by using natural products that are free from these compounds.

Formaldehyde

Formaldehyde is a commonly used preservative in cosmetics. Wait, hold up – isn't formaldehyde what they use to embalm bodies for funeral viewings? It can't be good to absorb that, right?

Formaldehyde is widely acknowledged to be a carcinogen, so why are cosmetic companies using it in their products? Formaldehyde is a very effective preservative, prolonging shelf life of products for years. No use-by date means no out-of-date products to dispose of, which greatly improves the bottom line of these huge corporations.

Formaldehyde in cosmetics usually comes from the use of formaldehyde-releasing chemicals. These chemicals silently release formaldehyde into the products as they sit on your shelves. You'll need to play a bit of detective work to find them, but they are:

- DMDM hydantoin
- Imidazolidinyl urea
- Diazolidinyl urea
- Quaternium-15
- Bronopol (2-bromo-2-nitropropane-1,3-diol)
- 5-Bromo-5-nitro-1,3-dioxane
- Hydroxymethylglycinate

As well as being associated with cancer, formaldehyde is also a skin irritant and has been associated with dermatitis. Obviously, avoiding these chemicals is a must.

Breast cancer donations from skin care companies

One of my pet hates is the way in which cosmetic companies advertise that they are 'joining the fight against cancer' by donating some of their profits to breast cancer research. This is highly hypocritical, considering that these companies are well aware that phthalates and parabens, ingredients which are in nearly every product they sell, cause cancer. Surely, if they wanted to make a real difference, they would remove these cancer-causing ingredients to prevent cancer, rather than claiming to help cure it? One study even found that high phthalate levels stopped chemotherapy from being as effective. I'm all for joining the fight against cancer, but we need to start from the ground up if we really want to eradicate this devastating disease.

Fragrance

'Fragrance' is a term that can be used to cover thousands of potential chemicals used in cosmetics and skin care. Labelling legislation allows for chemicals that make up a fragrance to be grouped and listed as 'fragrance' on the label.

Phthalates are a common inclusion in fragrance, as are hormone-disrupting octoxynols and nonoxynols. Fragrance may also contain the synthetic musks galaxolide and tonalide. These chemicals can stimulate your oestrogen receptors and have been shown to also affect androgen and progesterone receptors. Tonalide has also been reported to increase the proliferation of oestrogen-dependent breast cancer cells. A single fragrance can contain up to 200 different chemicals, many of which are harmful to your health.

The truth about fragrance

Fragrance = chemical cocktail that is so bad that they don't even want to list it on the label. At least the term 'fragrance' is easy to identify and therefore easy to avoid. Also beware of products marked as 'unscented' – this can just mean that there are chemicals to mask the scents in the product.

Dioxins

By now I hope that your conventional personal care items are already on their way to the bin, but if you're not yet convinced there is more. Dioxins are cancer-causing compounds that are created by ingredients such as polyethylene glycol (PEG), triclosan, emulsifiers and sodium laureth sulfate. Sodium laureth sulfate and sodium lauryl sulfate are also surfactants, which help the product to penetrate the skin more easily. This is bad news if they're in products which also have other nasty chemicals that are harmful to your health, as they can increase the amount that is absorbed dramatically.

Antiperspirants and deodorants

Antiperspirants pose two problems. First, they are a toxic blend of chemicals that can be absorbed straight into your bloodstream. Second, they stop the natural process of perspiration (sweating), which means you can't get your toxins out. So if they can't come out, where do you think they end up? In your body, of course.

Antiperspirants contain either aluminium or a chemical alternative which is likely worse for you than the aluminium was. They are also laced with 'fragrance' and other chemicals like parabens, as are deodorants. Interestingly, studies on breast cancer have found that the outer section of the breasts develops more tumours than the inner sections, and this has been thought to be due to the use of antiperspirants and deodorants. The mounting research on xenoestrogens like phthalates and parabens has launched an interesting series of discussions about what role these personal care products could have in breast cancer development.

You also need to avoid natural antiperspirants, like crystal based ones, which also contain aluminium and stop your natural perspiration. Go for a 100 per cent natural deodorant, free from 'fragrance' or chemical additives.

Cleaning chemicals

Cleaning products are another major source of toxins, and the more you use them, the more of the following toxins you're likely to be inhaling and absorbing through your skin.

Triclosan

This chemical is found in dishwashing detergents and antibacterial hand washes. It is an aggressive antibacterial that can promote the growth of nasty drug-resistant bacteria. We are exposed to thousands of bacteria every day – this is a normal part of living and helps to keep us balanced. However, agents like triclosan encourage resistance among these bacteria – not only to common household 'germs' but to also to conventional antibiotics that may be needed someday to save your life. Early studies also indicate that triclosan is an endocrine disruptor and it even impaired muscle function in mice.

So ditch your dishwashing liquid and use only natural hand wash and detergents to avoid this chemical. Triclosan can also be used in toothpaste and deodorant, so look out for it on the label.

Quaternary Ammonium Compounds (QUATs)

QUATs are found in liquid fabric softeners and most household cleaners that are listed as 'antibacterial'. Like triclosan, they pose the same problem with creating superbugs that are resistant to antibiotics. They are also linked to skin disorders and asthma development.

2-Butoxyethanol

2-Butoxyethanol is the key ingredient in window cleaners that gives them that characteristic sweet smell. It is a powerful solvent that, in high enough doses, can cause lung, liver and kidney problems. Use vinegar in a spray bottle instead as an easy option to avoid this cleaner.

Ammonia

Found in glass cleaner and polishing products, ammonia is a powerful irritant that causes asthma and breathing problems. Housekeepers nearly always develop breathing problems or asthma because of this chemical.

 TIP: *Bicarbonate of soda, lemon juice and vinegar have a long history of use for all kinds of cleaning tasks. Search online for natural home cleaning tips and tricks.*

Chlorine

As well as being found in tap water, chlorine is used in powerful cleaning products like mould removers, scouring powders, toilet cleaners and laundry whiteners. You absorb it through your skin but also through inhalation when cleaning with it. As well as disrupting your thyroid due to competing with iodine in the body, it can affect your breathing as well.

Perchloroethylene (PERC)
Used in dry cleaning, spot removers and carpet cleaners, PERC is a neurotoxin and possible carcinogen.

This list is just touching the surface. Your best bet is to substitute all cleaning products for natural alternatives. Steam cleaning is also a great way to remove grime without chemicals.

Major toxin sources

Food
Conventional food contains traces of pesticides containing xenoestrogens, which act as hormone disruptors in the body. Meat and dairy products are also a source of added hormones and antibiotics.

Water
Tap water can contain high levels of chlorine and fluoride – both of which can displace the important mineral iodine which is needed for thyroid health and breast health. Ground water can contain heavy metals and other environmental toxins like pesticide residue.

Rain water can also contain toxins due to it being collected from rooftops that are painted, and stored in plastic or metal tanks which can leach toxins into the water.

The lesson? Always filter your water, no matter the source.

Soil
Our soil is a reservoir for toxins – it can contain heavy metals like lead and residues of pesticides like DDT. Remember the former uses of many city parks and gardens. If you're suspect about your own soil then you may want to get it removed and start with some fresh soil from a nursery. You can then boost its nutrition with your own compost.

Air pollution

Our air quality deteriorates the closer we get to the city, but also if we are around mining areas that process the minerals nearby. Farming areas that crop spray are also a concentrated source of pesticides and fertilisers, which can be detrimental to your health. If you are driving, consider keeping the windows down when the air is clean and keep them up in heavy traffic to keep out fumes. Car fumes contain cadmium and formaldehyde, both of which you want to be avoiding.

Skin care

A concentrated source of parabens, phthalates and even formaldehyde, conventional skin care is one of the most detrimental products for your health.

Cleaning products

Cleaning products are a major source of toxins, especially if you are using them regularly. They contain phthalates, as discussed previously, and other nasties you want to be avoiding.

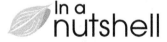 In a nutshell

You are a product of your environment, so make sure you observe what you're exposing yourself to every day. After reading this section you should have a clear idea of what kind of toxins are adding to your daily load. The next step is taking some action and changing your environment so that it can help your cells to heal and bring you one step closer to getting well and staying well.

PART 3

HOW TO FIX IT

*'If a fish is swimming in a dirty tank and it gets sick,
do you take it to the vet and amputate the fin? No, you
clean the water. By eating organic raw greens, nuts
and healthy fats, I am flooding my body with enzymes,
vitamins and oxygen.'*
              – KRIS CARR

So by now you're probably wondering how you can lessen the
impact these areas have on your life so you can get well and
stay well.

Some toxins can't be avoided, but many of them can.
Likewise, you might not be able to completely transform your life
right away, but you can certainly improve your body's ability to
cope with day-to-day stressors.

How?

1. **Clean up your diet**
   We have all heard the saying 'you are what you eat', so
   do you want to be fast, cheap and easy? Food is your
   body's fuel, and here you'll learn how to nourish your
   body so that it can perform at its peak.

2. **Give your body a spring clean**
   While cleaning up your diet is a long-term plan,
   sometimes your body needs a bit of extra help
   to cleanse. Regular detoxification is essential for
   anyone who lives in the modern world, experiences
   stress or eats any conventional food.

3. **Take time to unwind**

   Sleep and relaxation are essential for our bodies
   and minds – they give our bodies time to repair, and
   give our minds time to take a break from our day-
   to-day stressors.

4. **Move your body**

   Our bodies are designed to move, so it's time to get
   moving! You'd be surprised by just how much exercise
   can boost your mood as well as your overall health.

5. **Connect with nature**

   Numerous studies have shown how much the
   human body benefits from being in nature, both on
   a mental and cellular level. Here you'll learn more
   about the benefits, as well as how to get back to
   nature more often.

6. **Think healthy thoughts**

   Your mind controls your body, so a key element of
   getting well and staying well is thinking healthy thoughts.

7. **Ask for help**

   Even though there's a lot we can do on our own,
   sometimes we need a helping hand. Here you'll
   learn about the range of natural therapists who can
   assist you on your healing journey.

But, before we get started...

Before you start getting stuck into this section, I want you to
think about what you want for your health. After all, how can you
get where you want to go if you don't know where that is? The
most successful business people know that being clear about
your goals is essential for bringing them to life, and this is just
as true for your health, wellbeing and happiness goals.

So start by taking some time to think about your health
goals. How would you like things to be different six weeks from
now? How about six months from now? Be as specific as you can.

Once you have this picture, spend some time each day visualising yourself achieving it – what does it look like to truly be healthy? How does it feel? What will you be able to do or experience once you get well? Really immerse yourself in what it would be like to be where you want to be.

This goal will be your focus through the following chapters.

CHAPTER 7
DIET – YOU ARE WHAT YOU EAT

'Let food be thy medicine and medicine be thy food.'
– HIPPOCRATES

You are what you eat; so do you want to be cheap and easy, or bursting with goodness? As you know from Chapter 4, our modern diet isn't all it's cracked up to be. As a result, some of the things you took to be healthy are really not that great for you. That said, once you learn the simple rules behind eating healthily, you can enjoy a diet that is both nourishing and delicious, which is the first key to getting well and staying well.

You see, your body takes whatever it can from the fuel you put in it. Just think of what would happen to a high-performance race car if you used the lower-octane fuel that we use in our sedans. Would you get the most out of it?

Our bodies are no different – if we want to perform well then we need premium fuel. So what is the perfect diet to provide this premium fuel?

The perfect diet

With everyone touting their diet as the best, who should you believe? As a holistic naturopath, I know that there is actually no one diet that is perfect for every person. There are so many diets our there – low carb, vegan, paleo, FODMAPs, vegan, raw food etc. I'm not an advocate for any of these diets, although I have recommended each of them for certain clients at some point, and have tried them all out myself.

I don't believe that there is any one way of eating that suits every person, so you need to work out what is right for you. There will be foods you don't do well with, and there will be foods that your body thrives on. We are all individuals with different genetic makeups, different digestive capacities and different nutritional needs, which means the perfect diet for you will be different to the perfect diet for your partner or a sibling.

This means one person will be able to tolerate one food well while another may not be able to. This comes down to:

- Your digestive acid and enzyme capacity
- Your local tolerance to compounds in foods
- Your immune system and allergic response
- The health of the intestinal wall
- The health of the microbiome (i.e. good versus bad bacteria)

Food intolerance is extremely common due to our lifestyles – too much sugar, refined food, alcohol and trans fats and not enough fresh fruit and vegetables has led to an inability to digest as well as we used to. As I mentioned earlier, food isn't really food anymore either, and has become so incredibly processed that we can't tolerate it like we used to.

So how do you know what's right for you? Listen to your body. By now you should be getting a sense for what is normal and what is not. The easiest way to identify if a food is good for you or not is to notice how your body reacts to that food in a food challenge.

Food intolerance challenge

1. Stop eating the suspected food or food group for two weeks.
2. At the end of the two-week period, eat a couple of meals that are high in the food or ingredient you have been avoiding. For example, if you were avoiding wheat, then you might have a sandwich for lunch and pasta for dinner.
3. Observe any symptoms you experience – any bloating, indigestion, noisy digestion, burping, wind or bowel changes? Any fatigue or mood changes?

You are much more likely to notice food symptoms if you eliminate the food for a couple of weeks and then reintroduce it, because your body can adapt and try to 'cope' with the intolerance when it is eaten regularly.

If you react to some foods 'sometimes', then I recommend avoiding them too. Although they are only giving you noticeable symptoms some of the time, there is a good chance that they are causing a low-grade inflammation every time you eat them, even if you don't notice it. Food intolerance is usually a result of digestive dysfunction and imbalance. If you eliminate the food that is causing the problem, and do some digestive healing under the advice of a naturopath, there is a good chance that you'll be able to desensitise to the food and eat it here or there in the future without an issue.

Redefining 'diets'

The definition of diet is actually 'habitual food' or 'what you eat on an everyday basis'. You'll notice this isn't a short-term practice, it's about learning what works for your body over the long term.

A healthy diet will give you good nutrition, help you maintain a healthy weight, and provide what you need for energy and all of your body functions. A healthy diet doesn't have to be boring – in fact, it should be filled with varied, wholesome and delicious foods!

In this section I'm going to give you the rundown on what I perceive as the keys to an easy-to-follow, healthy and wholesome diet. In simple terms, I'm going to teach you what you need to include and what you need to avoid. There will be no counting calories, no stages of eating and nothing that you absolutely have to do.

As a general rule, though, you'll see that everything that I recommend is in its pure, wholefood form. As I mentioned before, this doesn't mean you need to be chewing on wheat berries; it means that if something is made from wheat it needs to be made from the whole grain, not parts of it. If you implement only one thing from this book, make it to stick to whole and unrefined foods as the basis of your diet and you'll be on your way to wellness.

Basic nutritional requirements

To survive we need micronutrients and macronutrients. Micronutrients are nutrients like vitamins and minerals, while macronutrients, or 'big' nutrients, are protein, fats and carbohydrates, which our bodies break down to make energy.

Mainstream nutrition breaks these into percentages that you should be consuming, and the number of calories you need each day. For most people these numbers are confusing, so I prefer to work with the following:

1. What needs to be in each meal?
2. How big is the serving size?
3. What helps keep a meal balanced?

What needs to be in each meal?

Each meal should have all of the three macronutrients – proteins, fats and carbohydrates.

Proteins

Proteins are the building blocks for every tissue in the body. Proteins are made up of amino acids, which are needed for everything, including mood regulation, digestion, wound healing, memory and concentration, energy production and hormonal health. Your body uses proteins every moment to communicate between cells in the body. Without enough protein we can become depressed, fatigued and our sleep may be impaired.

So it goes without saying that protein is essential. Protein should be an inclusion in all of your main meals, and a lot of your snacks too. Protein comes from meat, poultry, fish, seafood, eggs, legumes, whole grains, nuts and seeds. You'll also find trace amounts of protein in green leafy veggies and mushrooms. Consider the source of your protein, as this will impact the quality of the nutrients you're receiving. Some meats may be high in hormones due to different farming practises (especially chicken and eggs), while seafood can be contaminated with toxins. This is why I recommend eating organic where possible.

Protein for vegans/vegetarians

Vegans can easily get enough protein to sustain them from nuts and seeds, legumes and whole grains. Vegetarians can also eat eggs and dairy products. It is very important that vegans, and vegetarians who don't eat much dairy or eggs, eat all three of the plant-based food groups on a daily basis, as vegan protein sources do not contain all of the essential amino acids.

Because our bodies cannot make these essential amino acids, we must get them from the diet in order to survive. Legumes, whole grains and nuts/seeds each lack certain essential amino acids so you need to consume all three groups. Contrary to popular belief, you do not need to combine your vegetarian protein sources at every meal. As long as you are getting all three protein groups (nuts/seeds, legumes and whole grains) every day then you will absorb the full range of amino acids required to sustain you.

Protein sources

Vegetarian sources include nuts, seeds, legumes (lentils, chickpeas, beans, peas), and whole grains (brown rice, quinoa, spelt, khorasan, barley, millet, amaranth).

Animal sources include eggs, chicken, turkey, other poultry, beef, lamb, kangaroo, pork, fish, shellfish, molluscs, and dairy products.

 TIP: *Kangaroo meat is an excellent source of iron, protein and other nutrients, if you can get over eating Skippy. Kangaroo meat is also high in omega 3, being free-range (omega 3 is found mostly in wild animals that are running around in their natural state – more on this under Fats). It is also one of the most sustainable meats with the lowest number of toxins. Try using kangaroo mince in place of beef or try the steak cooked medium rare and served with veggies.*

Fats

Fat is an essential part of the diet and due consideration should be taken that we are including enough, not avoiding it. The key is to eat the right balance of fats so your body gets what it needs to function effectively.

Saturated fat can be consumed as long as it is from a healthy source – organic meat, organic butter, macadamias and coconut oil are ideal sources of saturated fats.

Polyunsaturated and monounsaturated fats come from plant sources like olive oil, nuts, seeds and other oils like rice bran or grape seed oil.

Trans fatty acids are made when a fat is exposed to heat or pressure. They can be formed in unstable oils during cooking, and are found in margarine and deep-fried foods, particular those cooked in oils high in polyunsaturated fats like canola oil, sunflower oil and 'vegetable' oil. More on this on page 64.

Vegetable oil

Vegetable oil, believe it or not, is not made from vegetables. It is a broad term that can be used to describe any oil that contains any of the following:

- Canola oil
- Soy oil
- Sunflower oil
- Cottonseed oil
- Safflower oil
- Palm oil
- Peanut oil

Vegetables oils are cheaply made using chemical extraction and should be avoided completely.

Omega 3, 6 and 9

Omega 3, 6 and 9 fatty acids are beneficial components of fat that we need to survive. For most people eating a western diet, omega 3 is the one that is most commonly deficient as omega 6 and 9 are found in abundance in plant-based oils, avocados, nuts and seeds that we commonly consume.

Omega 3 is found mostly in wild animals – that is ones that are running around in their natural state. Fish, particularly oily fish like sardines, salmon, mackerel and tuna, are high in omega

3. Game meats and kangaroo are also an excellent source of omega 3 as they are much more active than pasture-raised beef and lamb.

Vegetarian omega 3 can also be sourced from chia seeds, flaxseeds, walnuts and some algae. However, these sources do need to be converted into active omega 3 by your body and may not be enough if you are deficient, particularly if you have any inflammatory conditions like endometriosis, autoimmune disease or arthritis.

Healthy fat sources

- Avocado
- Egg yolks
- Raw nuts
- Raw seeds
- Olive oil (cold-pressed)
- Macadamia oil (cold-pressed)
- Avocado oil (cold-pressed)
- Coconut oil (cold-pressed)
- Organic butter
- Organic animal fats (small amounts)

Fat stability

One of the biggest mistakes we make is eating a lot of unstable and altered fat. Consuming rancid fat is detrimental to our health. Unstable fat such as vegetable oil can become oxidised easily, which leads to disruption in the way that it is used in the body. These rancid fats are consumed every day in the modern diet in the form of cooked canola oil, 'vegetable' oil and sunflower oil.

Vegetable oils did not form part of the human diet before the 1920s and there is mounting evidence to suggest that their widespread use is what has caused the increase in cardiovascular disease that we have today. This is due to the fact that these oils are unstable and are not suitable for cooking. This, coupled with the fact that our omega 3, 6 and 9 balance has been thrown off by eating too much of these oils, is probably the reason why we are more prone to heart attacks now than ever before.

Cottonseed oil, one of the most popular margarine and vegetable oil ingredients, has natural toxins (unrefined cottonseed oil is actually used as a pesticide, although the toxin gossypol is removed during refining). Cotton is also one of the most heavily sprayed crops so it is likely cottonseed oil has high amounts of pesticide residues.

Canola oil, which is widely touted as the healthiest oil of all, has been associated with many health problems. A high consumption of canola has been linked with vitamin E deficiency as well as growth retardation in animals.

Nuts and seeds also contain natural oils that can become bad. When you grind, cook or expose nuts and seeds to light, the oils quickly oxidise and become rancid. This is why walnuts and Brazil nuts often taste bitter – this is actually a sign of rancidity and they should not be consumed. The seeds that contain the most delicate oil of all are flaxseeds, which can become rancid within hours of pressing the oil or grinding the seeds and should only be consumed fresh.

LSA recipe

LSA is a ground meal of linseeds (flaxseeds), sunflower seeds and almonds. Never buy premade LSA – the natural oils will be rancid by the time it gets to you. In fact, the oil of flaxseeds is so volatile that it begins to degrade the moment you crack the shell.

Making your own LSA allows you to get the full benefit of the natural oils and omega 3 the flaxseed contains. It is also high in vitamin E, calcium, magnesium, iron and zinc.

In a coffee grinder, nut grinder or food processor, place equal amounts of whole raw linseeds, sunflower seeds and almonds. Grind until fine and store in an airtight glass jar in the fridge immediately. Keeps for up to two weeks.

Use your LSA on porridge, muesli, yoghurt and in smoothies.

How to incorporate fats in your diet

Use the right oils in cooking

Only stable fats should be used for cooking. Butter, ghee, palm oil (ethically sourced) and coconut oil are the only oils that should be subjected to high temperature cooking like frying and baking. This is because they have a high level of saturated fat which stops them from turning rancid during the cooking process.

You can use macadamia oil or rice bran oil for lower temperature cooking like light sautéing, frying at low temperatures or baking under 160 degrees Celsius.

Use only cold-pressed oils

All non-animal oils, regardless of type, should be cold-pressed. This means that they press the oil out without heat or chemicals. Unfortunately mass-produced oil is normally made using heat and chemical extraction, which can leave chemical residues and damage the oil.

Eating raw oils

Olive oil is an excellent addition to many meals after cooking. It can be drizzled on salads, risottos, pasta, meat, veggies and eggs after cooking for extra nutrition and flavour. You can also use macadamia oil and avocado oil in the same way. This is one of the best ways to up your intake of vitamin E.

The truth about margarine

Margarine is a chemical product made from unhealthy oils and loaded with artificial colours and flavours. Margarine is not a healthy butter substitute and should not be a part of a healthy diet.

Here's how it is made:
The process starts with cheap, poor quality, unstable oils like corn, canola, cottonseed, soy or safflower. These oils are already rancid from being extracted from their seeds using high temperature, high pressure and chemical extraction.

The last bit of oil is usually removed with hexane, a solvent known to cause cancer. Although this hexane is subsequently removed, traces of it are inevitably left behind.

The raw oils for making margarine are then steam cleaned. The high temperatures destroy any nutrients and antioxidants.

The oils are then mixed with finely ground nickel, a highly toxic substance that serves as a catalyst for the chemical reaction during the hydrogenation process. Other catalysts may be used, but these, too, are highly toxic. The oil and nickel mix is then put under high temperature and pressure in a reactor.

Hydrogen gas is introduced into the reactor. The high temperature and pressure, together with the presence of the nickel catalyst, causes hydrogen atoms to be forced into the oil molecules. This turns the oil from a liquid into a semi-solid substance. Trans fats are formed during this process.

The oil that comes out of the partial hydrogenation process is a smelly, lumpy, grey grease. To remove the lumps, emulsifiers – which are like soaps – are mixed in.

The oil is steam cleaned to remove the odour of chemicals. This step is called deodorisation and it involves high temperatures and high pressure once again, which removes most remaining nutrients. The oil is then bleached to get rid of the not-so-appealing grey colour.

Synthetic vitamins and artificial flavours are mixed in to give flavour and a nutritional profile. Beta-carotene is added to make the margarine yellow, as synthetic colouring is not allowed.

Finally, the margarine is promoted to the public as a health food – with the full endorsement of many scientists, doctors, dieticians and health authorities.

Want to know how butter is made?

1. Put cream in churner.
2. Churn until butter forms and liquid is separated.
3. Squeeze out remaining liquid.
4. Done!

Which would you prefer?

Carbohydrates

The most recent of evils, poor old carbohydrates have been under fire lately as the cause of many of our health problems. This is somewhat true – some carbs really do cause significant health issues so it is important to know which types to avoid and which to consume. Sugar is the simplest form of carbohydrate and ultimately is what most carbs get broken down into for use by the body. You can get complex and simple carbohydrates as well as fibre, which falls in the carbohydrate family.

We need carbohydrates to survive – they are an essential source of energy and essential to gut health, as long as you eat the right type. The largest source of carbohydrates in the modern diet is wheat – pasta, bread, pastry, crackers, cake and cookies are our main sources. Besides wheat, rice is the next biggest carb source, as well as fruit, fruit juice and added sugar.

Simple carbohydrates are the ones you want to avoid – they include sugar, refined wheat ('white' products), white rice, noodles, potato and most bread. Simple carbs give you a quick burst of energy, spike your blood sugar and then send it crashing again.

Complex carbohydrates include wholegrain products and legumes – they contain natural fibre that helps to give you a slow release of energy over time, which helps sustain healthy blood sugar levels and maintain energy. Complex carbs are things like brown rice, quinoa, legumes, wholegrain bread, oats and whole grains. Vegetables also contain varying levels of carbohydrates.

Fruit and sugar intake

I'm often asked if fruit is healthy because of its high sugar levels. I believe that fruit, eaten as a whole food, is metabolised well by the body due to the presence of fibre, which slows the absorption of the sugar in the fruit. Fruit juice, on the other hand, should be avoided as it is a concentrated form of sugar.

How much should we eat?

You need to include proteins, fats and carbohydrates in your diet every day. But how much do you include of each?

Protein

When looking at protein in main meals, a good guide is to eat a serving about the size and thickness of the palm of your hand. This is usually 100-150g meat, two eggs, half a cup of lentils or a handful of nuts. If you are having protein in your snacks then a good guide is three fingers' worth of nuts (in length and depth), one boiled egg or a quarter cup of legumes (such as hummus).

I recommend getting the bulk of your protein from vegetarian sources to avoid causing too much inflammation in the body, as meat protein is very acidic in nature. If you're a meat eater, a good balance would be one or two red meat meals per week (kangaroo is a great choice), two fish meals and perhaps one poultry meal per week. All other meals should be based around vegetarian proteins like eggs, legumes, nuts, seeds or whole grains. Remember to count leftovers and lunches as a meal as well – not just dinner.

Fat
Fats and oils should be an inclusion in most of your meals. Fats help to reduce the glycaemic load of a meal and are a great addition to carbohydrate-rich meals for this reason. Include nuts, seeds, avocado, olive oil, coconut oil and/or butter and organic animal fats like dairy and chicken skin regularly.

A healthy amount of fat for a day might include two eggs, half an avocado, one tablespoon of coconut oil, a small handful of nuts, one tablespoon of olive oil, a piece of salmon with the skin on and a few tablespoons of full-fat yoghurt. As long as you're not deep frying your food or eating foods with refined oil in them, you'll struggle to eat too much fat in a day.

Carbohydrates
Most food has small levels of carbohydrates so you don't have to eat the higher sources at every meal. Simple carbs like sugar and 'white' products, should be avoided, but complex carbs, including wholegrain products and legumes, can be included as part of a healthy diet one to three times per day. Fresh fruit should also be included – two serves per day is fine for most.

TIP: *When eating potatoes keep the skin on. It contains Lipoic acid, a powerful antioxidant which helps to metabolise the carbohydrates in the potato. If they are covered in dirt, simply scrub off under running water and use as usual!*

How big is the serving size?

Now that you know how much of each macronutrient you should be eating, how does that combine over your day? In other words, how much food should you be eating a day?

The answer for most people is: less than you are having now. Research shows that we eat way more than we need to, so there are very few people that need to be increasing their serving sizes. According to *Mindless Eating* by Brian Wansick, our plate sizes have been increasing and, with them, our serving sizes. In Brian's fascinating book, he outlines how his research has shown that we eat until we 'think' we are full, rather than when we are actually full. This means that the bigger the plate or cup, the more we will actually consume before we feel satisfied.

As a general rule, most people benefit from eating five small meals a day, rather than three big ones. This gives your body a steady stream of nutrients and energy without putting a huge load on the digestion all at once. I like using handfuls to determine amounts, as this helps to simplify things – if you're larger your hands are probably going to be bigger and you'll need more. If you have a small frame, your hands will be smaller and you'll need to eat less.

Here are some suggestions for serving sizes:

- Muesli – two handfuls with enough milk (or milk alternative) to just cover.
- Eggs – two eggs with one or two slices of toast.
- Salad – three handfuls of greens with a serve of protein the size and thickness of your palm.
- Steak – the size and thickness of your palm with three handfuls of steamed veggies.

- Nuts – snack on around three fingers' worth (length and thickness).

Tips to guide your meal sizes

I like to use general and easy terms that you can understand, rather than working with grams and cups which can be inaccurate due to the variations in our body sizes. Use these tips to guide your meal sizes:

- Buy smaller plates and bowls.
- Eat only a protein serving the size and thickness of the palm of your hand.
- Keep grain servings to a 'small handful'.
- Eat as many salads and veggies as you like – except potato.
- Eat some fat at every meal, as long as it's from a healthy source.
- Eat slowly, chewing your food until it is a paste before swallowing.
- Eat until you feel seventy per cent full.

What keeps a meal balanced?

Choosing a balanced meal isn't too difficult. Your main meals should always contain a source of protein and some good fats. Ideally every savoury meal should contain a couple of handfuls of vegetables of different varieties to give you a wide range of nutrients. If you are eating carbohydrates, they should be complex and accompanied by other proteins such as meat, eggs, legumes or nuts.

Avoid eating high-carbohydrate meals without any protein or fat to balance – this will spike your blood sugar temporarily before it crashes down again. Also avoid eating large amounts of meat without adequate fibre in the form of vegetables, a large salad or whole grains or you can risk constipation.

TIP: *Remember to chew your food very well, until it is a paste in your mouth, to start the digestive process and aid the release of enzymes. Also, avoid drinking large amounts of fluid with meals as this will water down your stomach acid and impair digestion.*

What about micronutrients?

Micronutrients are the business end of what our body needs to survive. Beyond proteins, fats and carbohydrates, they include vitamins, minerals, antioxidants and phytonutrients, and are essential to life.

There are many nutrition books out there that go into great detail about each of the vitamins and minerals we need and why. You don't have to get bogged down in the details of which food to eat to get which vitamin – if you follow a varied diet with plenty of foods from the *oh-yeah list* on pages 124 – 144, you will most likely be getting all of the vitamins and minerals you need. However, if you're interested in learning more about what various micronutrients can do, and where you can find them (this is particularly relevant if you want to target a certain health issue), refer to the micronutrient charts in the *Resources* section at the back of this book.

Essentially, what you need to know is that vitamins and minerals fuel the thousands of reactions that need to occur each moment for your body to work. Without adequate nutrition, your cells, tissues and organs begin to under function and, as a result, you will end up with imbalance and resulting disease.

As well as your vitamins and minerals, there are dozens of other nutrients that have been discovered to be essential to health, such as bioflavonoids and omega 3. This list is growing as more and more research is done on the breakdown of food and what it actually contains, and you can learn about some of the most important ones in the *Resources* section.

How do I know if I'm getting enough micronutrients?

A healthy diet that contains plentiful fruit, vegetables, nuts, seeds, legumes and whole grains will contain all the essential nutrients you need. But if you're missing any major food source, you can become deficient very quickly. Here are some of the common things people miss out on and the nutrient deficiencies that might come about as a result:

- If you don't eat any nuts or seeds, you could be deficient in minerals like calcium, magnesium and zinc. If you don't eat red meat *or* nuts and seeds, you'll likely be low in iron and zinc.
- If you don't eat many vegetables or whole grains, you may be low in B vitamins.
- If you don't eat any fish, seaweed or seafood, you'll be deficient in omega 3 and iodine.
- If you don't eat any butter or eggs and don't get much sun, you could be low in vitamin D.
- If you restrict fat in your diet, you'll be low in vitamin E, vitamin A and vitamin D.
- If you don't eat any legumes, you could be missing out on B vitamins and iron.
- If you don't eat any fresh fruit, you're missing out on vitamin C.
- If you only eat cooked food, you're missing out on a heap of vitamins that are damaged by heat, including vitamin C and B vitamins.
- If you don't eat any animal products, you can easily become deficient in vitamin B12.

There are also a few other factors that can make you deficient in nutrients:

- If you drink alcohol regularly you'll be deficient in vitamins A, D, E, B1, B2, B5, B12, folate, and selenium.
- If you take the oral contraceptive pill, you'll be low in B2, Vitamin C, magnesium and zinc.

- Pregnancy can reduce your levels of vitamins B1, B5, B6, B12, C, D, and E, folate, iron, magnesium, manganese, selenium and zinc. These deficiencies can persist post-partum if you don't get the right nutritional support.

How do you know if you're deficient?

As a naturopath I have all kinds of crafty ways to check if you're nutrient deficient. Here are some of my favourites:

- **Brittle nails** – Calcium or protein deficiency
- **White spots on your nails** – Zinc deficiency
- **Vertical (lengthways) ridges on your nails** – Silica deficiency
- **Dry skin** – Essential fatty acid (omega 3, 6, 9) deficiency
- **Poor night vision** – Vitamin A deficiency
- **Red spots on your tongue** – Calcium deficiency
- **Quivering tongue when you poke it out** – Magnesium deficiency
- **Cracks on the lips** – B vitamin deficiency
- **Bumps on the back of arms** – Vitamin A deficiency

Essentially, you need to listen to your body. Beyond the symptoms listed above, go through the various symptoms and systems in *Part 1 – Know your body*. If something isn't running properly, there's a good chance you might be missing something.

The other thing to keep in mind is that there are several factors that reduce vitamins in the body, like drinking alcohol, smoking, certain medications and organ dysfunction, which can lower levels of your essential nutrients. Use the charts in the *Resources* section to check your intake – if you're not eating any of the major sources indicated or if you tick any of the 'things that reduce levels' boxes, you may need to up your intake.

The oh-yeah list – foods to eat heaps of

While you know you need your macronutrients and micronutrients, now you might be asking, 'So what should I actually eat? Which foods do I buy each week?'

There are plenty of foods that will help you sustain good health. These are your oh-yeah, eat-as-much-as-you-damn-please foods.

Green leafy veggies

Ever been told to 'eat your greens'? I hope you did, because these leafy wonders are the ultimate super food. Including the likes of spinach, kale, silver beet (chard), rocket, dark lettuce and beetroot tops, green leafy veggies have more health-giving effects than any other food. They boost nutrition, detoxify and alkalise the body. They are essential to life.

Properties of green leafy vegetables:

- **Alkalise the body** – This helps to reduce inflammation.
- **Help you detoxify** – The sulphur and chlorophyll binds to toxins to be excreted by the body.
- **High mineral content** – Leafy greens are a substantial source of iron, calcium and magnesium.
- **High antioxidant content** – Source of vitamin A and other antioxidants.
- **High fibre** – This further helps you expel toxins.

Greens should be eaten every single day – the more the better. Always use baby spinach, rocket or dark greens in salad (not iceberg lettuce, which is nutritionally void), add chopped or frozen spinach to curries, soups, quiches, stir fries and casseroles, and have some raw or sautéed greens on the side of any meal to increase intake. You can even try a green smoothie to boost your daily intake.

Green smoothies

A green smoothie is a great way to get in your daily dose of green leafy veggies. As well as being tasty and easy, having your greens blended breaks down the cellulose and cell walls much better than chewing, allowing you to get the maximum benefit from the greens.

You'll need a good blender for this – I use a Vitamix but any high-speed blender will do. If you have a crappy blender then use only soft fruits and baby spinach to begin with.

Basic green smoothie recipe
2 serves of fruit – bananas, berries, oranges, apples, watermelon, pineapple, kiwifruit – anything really.

1-2 handfuls of greens – try kale or baby spinach to begin with, but you can use any greens.

Water

Optional extras
Chia seeds or flaxseeds (pre-soaked are best)

Maca powder, cacao powder, spirulina or other super food powders

Cashews (to make it creamy – soak them first if you have a weaker blender)

For those who are more hard-core, you can also make a green smoothie with vegetables like cucumber, celery or tomato in place of the fruit.

Cruciferous vegetables

Cruciferous vegetables are made up of all of your childhood favourites – Brussels sprouts, cabbage, broccoli, cauliflower, radish, kale, bok choy and rocket (arugula). This gorgeous family of vegetables have been studied extensively and their intake has been linked to reduced rates of cancer and endometriosis.

Properties of cruciferous vegetables:

- **Detoxifying** – They contain indoles and sulphur compounds which help our body to detoxify excess hormones and environmental pollutants.
- **Anti-inflammatory** – they help to reduce inflammation in the body, which is essential to prevent disease.

Cruciferous veggies should be eaten every day. They are best taken lightly steamed or added in the later stages of cooking to preserve nutrients. You can also eat them raw. Caution must be taken for those with thyroid issues as cruciferous veggies contain goitrogens, which can cause an enlargement of the thyroid gland for people who are iodine deficient or are prone to thyroid dysfunction.

Sauerkraut – the ultimate health food

Sauerkraut is made from fermented cabbages. Not only does it give you the benefit of natural probiotics to improve gut health and immunity, it also is a good source of indoles and sulphur compounds, which can prevent cancer and help with hormonal health. Plus, it is super easy to make.

Ingredients

1 large cabbage with the outer leaves (you'll need around 2kg of cabbage).

3 tbsp Celtic sea or Himalayan salt.

Special equipment

A very large crock pot with a plate to weigh down your ingredients, or a special sauerkraut vessel. You could also use a large food-grade bucket with a plate that fits snugly inside.

Method

1. Chop cabbage finely or coarsely, depending how you'd like it. Place the cabbage in a large bowl as you chop it.

2. Sprinkle salt on the cabbage as you put it in the bowl. The salt is what will create the brine in which the cabbage will ferment without rotting. It also keeps the cabbage crunchy. Use more salt in summer and less in winter when spoiling is less likely.

3. Mix the cabbage and salt together and place in a crock or bucket. Pack a little in at a time, using your fists or a potato masher to press it down firmly. This helps to pack it down and encourage water to seep from the cabbage.

4. Cover sauerkraut with a plate or some other lid that will fit snugly inside the vessel. Place a clean weight (like a glass jar filled with water) on the cover to force water out of the cabbage and keep the cabbage submerged under the brine. Cover the top with a cloth tied on to keep flies out.

5. Press down on the weight to help force the water out of the cabbage. Continue doing this every few hours until the brine rises above the plate/cover. This can take around 24 hours. Older cabbage may contain less water and might take longer.

6. If the brine doesn't rise above the plate by the following day, add enough salted water to cover it (1 tbsp of salt to 1 cup of water).

7. Leave the cabbage to ferment. Check it every day or two. The volume will reduce as it ferments. Occasionally mould will appear on the top. Simply skim off what you can. The sauerkraut is still fine under the brine.

8. Rinse off the weight and the plate and taste the sauerkraut. It should be tangy after a few days and the taste will intensify as time passes. In cool weather it can ferment for months but in summer the process is much more rapid. It should become soft and the flavour will be pleasant.

9. The sauerkraut is now ready to eat! You can scoop some out and put it in a clean jar in the fridge and leave some still fermenting for a while if it is convenient, but make sure you repack it carefully.

10. Sauerkraut can keep in the fridge in brine for months, just be sure to use a clean spoon to get it out of the jar to prevent contamination.

Fruit

It goes without saying that fruit is healthy, but you'd be surprised by how many people neglect this important part of their diet. The fact is that you will get from fruit what no vegetable will give you – a different set of nutrients and fibre content. Fresh fruit is the best source of vitamin C and, for those that don't eat any raw veggies, likely their only source of vitamin C.

Of course different fruit has different properties and benefits, so ensure you're eating a variety to get broader health benefits. Just look at the following:

- Apricots are a rich source of iron.
- Figs and dates trump milk for calcium.
- Pawpaws and pineapples are anti-allergic.
- Tomatoes and watermelon contain lycopene, which protects your heart.

Want to know more? I've included a list of interesting fruit facts for you in the *Resources* section. Once you read it you'll see that if you want to prevent cancer and chronic disease, regular fruit intake is a must.

A note on dried fruit

The nutritional value of dried fruits depends on how they were dried – some drying techniques use heat which can destroy some nutrients. Organic and preservative-free dried fruit may be a useful addition to the diet – dates and figs are great for fibre and calcium and prunes are great for digestion. However, only eat as much dried fruit as you would fresh and count it towards your daily fruit intake.

Vegetables

You didn't need to read this book to know that you should be eating more vegetables – but it's an important message that most people don't put enough value on. Vegetables contain a wide spectrum of nutrients. Not only do they contain vitamins and minerals, they are rich and complex in phytonutrients that keep our cells working at their best.

Besides potato and corn, you can't really overdose on vegetables. Essentially, the more you eat, the better the health benefits. Aim to make at least fifty per cent of your food intake from vegetables and salads and your body will thank you.

Each vegetable has its own unique properties, many of which I have listed in the *Resources* section. To name just a few:

- Broccoli is a cancer-fighting cruciferous vegetable, high in calcium, folate and vitamin C. Bam!
- Asparagus can balance your blood sugar.
- Celery cleanses the kidneys.
- Peas and carrots help eye sight.
- Mushrooms can boost your immune system.

You can start to see that if you include a wide range of vegetables in the diet you'll be covered for most diseases. That's why your grandma always made you eat your veggies!

Herbs and spice and all things nice

Herbs and spices do so much more than give our food flavour. They are rich sources of nutrients and phytochemicals that have wide-ranging health effects.

Herbs and spices are aromatic in nature, and often contain high levels of essential oils which are healing, prevent oxidative damage to the body and can even help to control the overgrowth of bacteria in the gut. In fact, in India where spices like turmeric, cardamom, garlic and ginger are consumed with most meals, the rates of diabetes are just as high as in the west due to their rising intake of sugar. However, the rate of diabetic complications such as neuropathy, loss of vision, kidney disease and ulceration are much lower. This could be due to the fact that they consume large amounts of these aromatic spices, which have a powerful effect on circulation and can help to prevent oxidative damage in the body.

To name just a few, look what benefits you'll gain from spicing up your life:

- Ginger is anti-inflammatory and helps to improve circulation.
- Basil and parsley are excellent sources of iron.
- Mustard is great for sinus congestion and allergies.
- Turmeric is a superfood in its own right, being very anti-inflammatory, circulation boosting and detoxifying.

To learn more about the awesome properties of common herbs and spices, visit the *Resources* section.

Garlic – the great disease preventer

Garlic is prized by herbalists for its unique health-giving properties. It has been studied extensively and found to be have the following benefits:

- Reduces blood pressure and protects against cardiovascular disease
- Antiviral and immune enhancing properties
- Antibacterial and antifungal – can help to balance gut flora
- Prevents blood clots
- Improves circulation
- Helps with detoxification

Note: Eat raw, freshly crushed/grated garlic for the best benefit on gut health.

I recommend adding fresh and dried herbs, spices and aromatics to your meals frequently to boost your phytonutrient intake and prevent disease. Growing your own herb garden is a cost-effective and rewarding way to have these super foods on hand to put in your meals.

Legumes

Legumes, or pulses, include lentils, beans and chickpeas. This food family is eaten all over the world as a cheap and excellent source of protein. Not only are legumes high in protein, but they are also one of the best sources of soluble fibre. Soluble fibre is needed to 'feed' the good bacteria in the gut, where it acts as a prebiotic. Prebiotics are important to keep your microbiome (gut flora) healthy, to balance blood sugar and to help with detoxification. Legumes also have hormone-balancing properties as they contain phytoestrogens.

Legumes are an ideal base for meals and I recommend that they be consumed regularly. However, they need to be prepared properly to remove a compound called saponins from the outside of their skins. Saponins can irritate the gut and cause problems like bloating and wind, particularly for those with weaker digestive systems. Legumes also have a high fibre content which can further irritate the digestion for those who don't break them down properly. If legumes upset your digestion, then see a naturopath for help or stick to more easily digestible legumes like borlotti beans, black-eyed beans and split red lentils.

Legumes are also a great source of iron (especially chickpeas and lentils), B vitamins and other trace minerals.

Preparing legumes

Preparing legumes properly is essential to allow for proper digestibility.

Step 1 – Soaking

All whole legumes need to be pre-soaked. The soaking process helps to hydrate the dried legume and remove some of the saponins (a phytochemical that causes gut irritation). You'll see the saponins as a 'soapy' appearance in the water when you rinse them. As legumes differ in their size and density there are different soaking times for each; however, a good guide is to soak them for at least twelve hours, or overnight.

Note: Add some wakame to the soaking and cooking water to help to soften the legumes.

Step 2 – Rinsing

After soaking, discard the water and rinse well. Put legumes in a large saucepan with plenty of water (at least three times as much water as the legumes).

Step 3 – Cooking

To cook legumes, bring to the boil then reduce heat to a low boil. Cooking times for legumes vary, with some only needing forty-five minutes and others needing several hours. Use the guide below for different legume types, or cook until tender.

Note: Don't add salt to the cooking water! It retards the skins – add it after cooking.

Legume type	Cooking time
Adzuki beans	50 – 60 minutes
Black beans	60 – 90 minutes
Black eyed peas	50 – 60 minutes
Borlotti beans	45 – 60 minutes
Cannellini beans	45 – 60 minutes
Fava beans (without skin)	50 – 60 minutes
Chickpeas	2 – 3 hours
Kidney beans	1 ½ – 2 hours
Brown lentils	45 – 75 minutes
Green lentils	30 – 50 minutes
Lima beans	60 – 90 minutes
Mung beans	60 – 75 minutes
Navy beans	50 – 60 minutes
Pinto beans	60 – 90 minutes

Step 4 – Rinsing and serving

Once the legumes are soft, take them off the heat and let them cool for five to ten minutes. Drain and rinse well under running water.

How to enjoy legumes

- Chickpea or lentil salad with chopped parsley, roast pumpkin and baby spinach
- Blend legumes with olive oil and spices for a delicious dip
- Use them in curries
- Cook them with onion and tomato and have them on toast for breakfast
- Make a soup or stew with them
- Use them in place of meat protein in salads, stews and casseroles

 TIP: *Because legumes take a while to cook, I recommend making them in large batches and then storing them in the fridge or freezer for later use.*

Nuts and seeds

Nuts and seeds are a great source of protein, fibre and the good fats that are essential to health. These good fats help nourish your cells, improve hormonal balance and keep your skin supple. Nuts and seeds are also a great source of minerals – eating a variety of raw nuts and seeds will boost your intake of iron, calcium, magnesium and zinc.

Check out these amazing benefits that you'll go nuts for!

- Brazil nuts are a rich source of selenium, which is needed for thyroid health and to detoxify the body
- Chia seeds and flaxseeds both contain vegetarian omega 3 and have prebiotic qualities, helping to feed your good gut bacteria
- Pepitas are one of the best sources of zinc
- Sunflower seeds have more iron, kilo for kilo, than red meat!

To learn more about the benefits of different nuts and seeds, refer to the *Resources* section.

Nuts and seeds should only be consumed raw as cooking destroys the good oils that they contain. Soaking (activating) your nuts will help to unlock their nutritional potential and make them easier to digest.

Almond milk

Almond milk is an excellent dairy alternative. It's a great source of calcium and the only milk that is alkaline. Homemade is much better than the store-bought ones, which are heat treated and usually contain sugar.

How to make almond milk

Soak 1 cup of almonds overnight in filtered water.

Discard water in the morning and rinse well.

Put in blender with 3 cups of water, a pinch of Himalayan or Celtic sea salt, and 1 tbsp cold-pressed macadamia oil or avocado oil.

Blend for 1-3 minutes, depending on how powerful your blender is.

Drain through a nut milk bag and store in the fridge for up to three days.

 TIP: *Use leftover nut meal in patties or to thicken soups. You may like to keep the fibre in and just shake it through before use if you're using your almond milk in smoothies or on muesli.*

Supercharged super foods

Super foods are foods that have particularly high levels of nutrients that can boost our health. I've mentioned that there are many day-to-day foods that we eat that have super food properties like broccoli, flaxseeds, turmeric and garlic.

There are also foods that you can buy as additives to the diet. You can eat these super foods to many different ways – often an easy way is to add them to smoothies, muesli or bliss balls.

Some of my favourite super foods are:

- Bee pollen – immune enhancing, antiviral and loaded with vitamins and minerals
- Chlorella – an algae that is an amazing detoxifier
- Cacao – high in magnesium, B vitamins and mood boosting theobromine
- Green tea – shown in studies to fight cancer, improve gut bacteria, prevent diabetes and have antioxidant effects
- Maca – this Peruvian super food is great for the your endocrine system and hormonal balance

Learn more about these foods and their amazing health benefits in the *Resources* section.

Coconut – the ultimate superfood

Water, oil, everything! Coconuts are one of the most amazing foods on Earth. Any part of the coconut is beneficial for health, but here is what each part does for us:

- Coconut water – A healthy, cleansing drink. It is found in young coconuts before the flesh develops. Coconut water is nature's sports drink – it is full of electrolytes that help hydrate your cells and provide fluid balance in the body. Interestingly, coconut water is so similar in makeup to human plasma that it was used as a transfusion during World War Two. Drink during and after sports and exercise, and while drinking alcohol and the next day to prevent a hangover.

- Coconut oil – The oil is made from the flesh of the coconut and has an ideal blend of healthy fats. It is high in Lauric acid, which exerts antifungal, antibacterial and antiviral effects. The fats in coconut oil are metabolised quickly in the body and are much less likely to be stored as fat. This makes it an ideal fat for weight management. It is a very stable oil that can be used in cooking without risking damage to its structure.

- Coconut milk – Coconut milk has some of the properties of coconut oil. It is also a good source of fibre, B vitamins and vitamin E. The canned variety does contain BPA, though, so don't consume too much of this.

Super food bliss balls

Bliss balls are a great sweet treat. They are packed full of nutrition so are great for snacking to boost your nutritional intake.

Coconut and goji berry bliss balls

Ingredients:

½ cup goji berries

½ cup raisins

½ cup warm water

1 cup raw cashews

½ cup coconut

1 tbsp unhulled tahini

1 tbsp chlorella powder or another super food powder

How to make them:

1. Place goji berries and raisins in a bowl with the warm water and mix through. Leave for fifteen minutes, stirring occasionally.
2. Meanwhile, process cashews on low in a food processor until chopped finely. Remove from processor and place aside.
3. Place soaked goji berries and raisins in the food processor with soaking water. Process into a paste.
4. Add cashews, coconut, tahini and chlorella to processor. Process on medium until well combined.
5. Roll into balls and toss in shredded coconut.
6. Store in the fridge for up to two weeks.

Cure-alls

There are many super foods that are touted to cure just about anything. It seems that as soon as some new food is discovered, there is a bandwagon of marketers out there to make a buck on selling it on its merits. Many of these super foods do have amazing health benefits, but so does an organic tomato for goodness sake. These foods are often awesome for you as part of a nutritious diet but there is no 'cure all', so beware of misleading claims.

Fermented foods

Eating fermented foods is one of the very best things that you can do for your health. There are lots of research papers on probiotics and probiotic foods and what they do for us.

They can help our immune system, prevent allergies, improve our moods and enhance digestion. Including varied probiotic foods in the diet helps to give you a constant supply of these health-giving probiotics, and will save you a heap on expensive probiotic supplements.

Try to include a couple of different types of probiotic foods to get a wide range of friendly bacteria. Avoid probiotic foods that are laden with sugar (like Yakult and many pre-packaged foods) as the sugar content can cause an overgrowth of 'bad' organisms which defies the purpose of eating the fermented food.

Yoghurt and fermented dairy

Yoghurt and fermented dairy products have been used across many cultures (no pun intended) for thousands of years. Unfortunately, most of the low-fat, sweetened 'yoghurts' that we get at the supermarket contain little to no probiotics and are detrimental to your health. When buying your yoghurt, look for ones that are tub set and have active probiotics without sugar. Or, better still, make your own.

You can make your own dairy yoghurt by using special yoghurt-making probiotics which are available at health food stores or perhaps through your naturopath (we sell them to our patients). You can also make yoghurt by using yoghurt – the cultures already present will multiply to give you more yoghurt and so on and so on.

Dairy intolerant? You can also make yoghurt out of coconut milk and other milk alternatives, if you're creative and willing to experiment a bit. Fermentation of alternative milk varies depending on the nutritional content as bacteria feed on the sugars and protein in the milk. A favourite of mine is cashew yoghurt, which is super easy to make and delicious too!

You can also get fermented cheeses like quark, which are very nutritious and also a great source of probiotics.

Cashew yoghurt

Cashews have naturally occurring bacteria on the outside which will ferment in the right conditions to make delicious yoghurt. You can also try this in combination with other nuts or chia seeds added for extra nutrition.

1. Place raw cashews and water in a blender.
2. Blend until smooth.
3. Cover with a clean towel and leave overnight to ferment, or longer if you live in a cold climate.
4. Voila! Your yoghurt is ready to eat. It only lasts a few days in the fridge so eat it up quickly.

Serve with fresh fruit, on muesli, in smoothies or on its own for a tasty snack.

Kefir

Kefir is a fermented drink made with kefir 'grains', which are really just colonies of the bacteria. You can make kefir on water or milk. The 'mother' culture can be found in some health food shops or by asking around. Facebook groups around fermenting foods are a great place to connect with other people and share cultures.

Kombucha

Kombucha is a drink like kefir but is usually made on tea. You can buy kombucha at some health food shops but it is far more economical to make your own. Again, look for the culture through online groups.

Sauerkraut and fermented vegetables

Sauerkraut (for recipe see page 126) and fermented vegetables like kim chi are a fantastic way to get a regular intake of friendly bacteria. However, most of the canned and jarred varieties do not contain this bacteria due to the heating (pasteurisation) process. If you are buying fermented vegetables, be sure to make sure that they are raw and unpasteurised to maintain good levels of healthy bacteria.

This information just touches on the wide variety of cultured foods that are available. To learn further, I recommend reading *Wild Fermentation* by Sandor Ellix Katz, which is packed with recipes to ferment all kinds of wonderful things.

Taking probiotics

A probiotic supplement can be a good addition to help your health but will never replace a healthy microbiome, which is made up of thousands of different microbes each with varying roles. Taking a probiotic when you have an imbalance in the microbiome is like pouring them into a pot of acid – although it won't harm you, the bacteria will not survive well in your gut like this. A better option is to see a naturopath and complete a gastrointestinal detox program which will help to kill off bad bacteria and then include probiotics so that in the end you end up with a healthier microbiome, rather than just wasting money on ongoing probiotic therapy. If you *are* taking a probiotic, look for one with multiple strains. Probiotics which are kept in the fridge are preferable to shelf-stable ones.

Too much of a good thing

Although these foods can be healthy at times, any food can cause health problems when eaten in excess. A balanced and varied diet is the best thing to ensure a wide range of different nutrients. There are, however, a few foods which you should limit your intake of to keep your health in check.

Fruit

Fruit contains sugars, which are fine when consumed in their natural, wholefood form, but even then you can have too much. Keep your fruit intake to two to three serves per day – a serve being around the size of an apple. You might, for instance, have one apple and three apricots or a small handful of grapes. If eating dried fruit, eat as much as you would if it were fresh – for example, you might eat three apricots in a sitting so three dried apricots would be fine. If you are eating a Palaeolithic or grain-free diet then you can allow for three to four serves of fruit as you will be getting fewer carbohydrates elsewhere.

Grains

As a general rule I like to encourage my clients to eat at least one grain-free meal each day. When you do eat grains, try to mix them up a bit rather than eating the same grains at every meal.

Wheat

No matter how organic, fermented or fine you are with wheat, I'd still recommend keeping it to one serve per day, if you choose to eat it at all.

Dairy

Keep dairy intake to a minimum – for most people I recommend one serve of organic yoghurt or cheese up to four days per week, if it is right for your body.

Red meat

Red meat, if from an organic, pasture-fed source, contains many vitamins and minerals and is a great source of protein. However, studies covering many different conditions all come to the same conclusion – a high intake of red meat causes disease. I'd recommend keeping red meat to a maximum of two serves per week – and this includes lunches *and* dinners.

Water

You can over hydrate! Drinking large amounts of water can leach the minerals from your body and put too much pressure on the kidneys. If you're super thirsty, it might be time to see your GP or naturopath to check it out.

 TIP: *Calculate your individual water requirements using this equation:*

Your weight in kg x .033 = litres of water you need per day.

You'll need to increase this if you're exercising or sweating a lot.

Do I have to be healthy all the time?

While I'm hoping that this chapter has got you excited about all of the delicious, healthy foods you can add to your diet, sometimes it can feel like there's no time for fun.

This isn't designed to be a short-term fix, but a long-term plan to achieve balance. And you can't have balance if you don't get to enjoy the things you love, even if those things include treats like wine, chocolate and coffee. So my goal isn't for you to cut these foods out entirely, but for you to eat amazingly ninety per cent of the time so that the ten per cent of the time doesn't really matter as much.

So how can you have your cake and eat it too? Let's explore some common 'treats' and see where they fit in to the health picture.

Alcohol

Alcohol, when taken in excessive amounts or the wrong type, is quite detrimental to your health. But included in moderate amounts as part of a healthy diet, it should not cause a problem.

I don't recommend drinking spirits with any type of soft drink, because drinking these easy-to-down beverages can lead to high alcohol consumption. I do think, however, that small amounts of spirits on the rocks or with soda water and lime are okay every now and then, as long as you keep your intake to a minimum (more on this in a few paragraphs).

Beer is high in yeast, so isn't something that I recommend that you drink too regularly as it can mess with your gut flora. Again, small amounts of preservative-free beers can be fine in moderation. Look for gluten-free beer if you are avoiding gluten, though.

Wine is one of the purest forms of alcohol, particularly if you can get it preservative-free. Red wine is always going to trump white due to the health benefits associated with resveratrol, which comes from the grape skins that it is fermented with.

As part of your regular diet, I'd recommend drinking no more than once or twice per week, with a maximum of two to three drinks at a time. Make it a red wine, or a vodka with fresh lime and soda if possible, or perhaps a couple of preservative-free beers.

Hangover prevention

When you get severely intoxicated, it actually damages your cells, and this is what gives you the hangover. Binge drinking is not something you should be doing regularly if you want to have good health. But, let's face it – there will always be that wedding, that party or that special occasion where you may get a little tipsier than usual. Even naturopaths like to let their hair out sometimes, and this is how you can help to mitigate the damage caused:

1. Stay hydrated

Half the problem with hangovers is that your cells are so severely dehydrated it is causing them to die. Make sure you drink well the day before the occasion, and have a glass of water after every alcoholic beverage. Have a huge drink of water before you pass out in bed.

2. Slow it down

Avoid having drinks quickly in succession. Using the tip above will help with this.

3. Drink coconut water

Coconut water is rich in the electrolytes that are needed to hydrate your cells, so drink before, during and after consuming alcohol. Keep in the fridge for the day after for a rescue drink, too.

4. Eat

Make sure you eat! Having food in your tummy helps to soak up some of that alcohol and slow down the absorption so it doesn't go straight to your head.

5. Try not to go over six drinks in one sitting

Try not to get to the point where you can't count where you're up to!

6. Take a B vitamin prior to drinking

This will help reduce your depletion and prevent hangover blues.

7. Have some grapefruit or tart orange juice ready for the morning

This will stimulate your liver to flush out the toxins from the night before.

Hangover cure drink

Got a hangover? Try this amazing pick me up that will soothe your woes:

150ml coconut water

150ml orange or grapefruit juice

Pinch Celtic sea salt

Mix together and drink liberally to rehydrate.

Coffee – friend or foe?

Coffee can be a friend or foe when it comes to your health. A moderate intake of coffee, say one to two cups per day (that's standard cups, not mugs or double shots) can be great for your health. Go above this, though, and we're talking about some serious health problems.

Coffee contains antioxidants and nutrients that can help your health. It may help improve memory and cognitive function, boost your metabolism and help you burn fat. Coffee can improve performance when exercising, reduce your risk of diabetes, protect against Alzheimer's and dementia and prevent cardiovascular disease.

A higher intake of coffee, however, can lead to anxiety, increased blood pressure, adrenal exhaustion and can aggravate migraines, arrhythmias and cause sleep disturbance. And four or more cups a day is associated with an increased risk of death, according to one Harvard study.

In my experience, I have found that those with sleep issues, fatigue or adrenal depletion benefit from taking a 'coffee break' for a few weeks or more to allow their adrenal glands to repair. This will mean that the body is much better able to deal with the effect of the caffeine from the coffee. For general health I recommend no more than one cup of coffee a day, in the morning, with one day a week coffee free. Drink only brewed coffee, never instant (which contains chemical residues from processing). Only drink coffee in the morning when cortisol is naturally high as caffeine consumption later in the day can cause problems with your sleep/wake cycle.

Decaf coffee

Decaf coffee is an option for those who are sensitive to caffeine. Use only Swiss water decaffeinated coffee – others are made with chemicals to strip the caffeine from the coffee beans.

Tea

Tea is worth a mention as, although it is a better option than coffee, it is still a source of caffeine and needs to be taken in moderation. I have on occasion come across patients that drink black tea all day long. When you are having tea in these quantities you'll get the same detrimental effects of coffee due to the caffeine content. A cup of tea contains around one-third of the amount of caffeine as a cup of coffee.

Tea and coffee are also acid-forming, leading to more inflammation in the body. Keep to two to three cups a day. Also be wary of added sugar you may be consuming with any tea or coffee intake.

Green tea is a much healthier alternative to black tea, being higher in antioxidants and less acidic in the body. Drink up to four cups a day but not in the evening, as it contains the same amount of caffeine as black tea.

It's all from the same bush

Green tea, black tea and white tea all come from the same plant, camellia sinensis. Black tea is made by steaming and fermenting the leaves. Green tea is made by fermenting the raw leaves and white tea has the most antioxidants of all, being made from the young tips of the tea plant.

Rooibos tea

Rooibos tea, or South African Bush Tea, is an excellent tea alternative. It is free from caffeine, has no tannins (which can inhibit mineral absorption), and is also loaded with beneficial antioxidants. Drink up!

Treating yourself – cakes, sugar and all things nice

'So, how much chocolate can I have?' Donna asked me one day.

There are some things that you just love and don't want to give up in the quest for pure, amazing health. You'll be pleased to know that you don't have to. Well, not completely, anyway.

It is really important to keep 'treats' to a minimum, but if I had to put a limit I'd say once per week might be okay to treat yourself to that piece of cake or chocolate. If you have a healthier option available – like dark chocolate over milk, or a cake made with xylitol instead of sugar – you'll be better off for it in the long run and may be able to have the foods you love a little more often.

Healthy sugar substitutes

For those with a sweet tooth, there are a lot of healthier alternatives to sugar. For most people the use of these substitutes can be part of a healthy diet and can really help those that are reducing sugar to ease the transition.

Honey – Honey is a natural whole food and has a lot of health benefits. Raw, unfiltered honey is a source of B vitamins and can boost your immune system. Honey is generally well tolerated by diabetics and is much more pancreas-friendly than sugar.

Maple syrup – Another whole food, maple syrup is made by tapping the bark of a maple tree. Maple syrup is a source of trace minerals and can be used in small amounts as part of a healthy diet.

Coconut sugar – Coconut sugar is derived from coconut palm blossoms. It is has a much lower GI than sugar (35 compared to sugar which has a GI of 68) and tastes a bit like brown sugar. It is also a source of minerals.

Dates – Dates are an excellent natural sweetener that can be used in baking, smoothies and treats for a natural sweetness that is also high in calcium and fibre.

Xylitol – A favourite of mine for baking substitution, xylitol is a natural fruit sugar that is very low GI and not well-absorbed by the gastrointestinal tract. It is low in calories and tastes just like sugar. Xylitol can also prevent tooth decay.

Stevia – Stevia is a natural herb that is extremely sweet. It is a sugar substitute that is practically calorie free and can be used as an alternative to sugar and artificial sweeteners. Look for natural stevia extracts, not heavily processed ones.

Agave – healthy or not?

Agave used to be touted as a healthy and 'raw' alternative to sugar, until it was discovered that it had similarities to high fructose corn syrup. It's probably best to avoid this sugar substitute and stick to honey or maple syrup.

Guilt-free 10-minute chocolate

This is a great recipe for when you really need some chocolate quick smart but are trying to maintain a healthy lifestyle. The coconut oil provides awesome fats and the cacao powder is a great source of calcium and magnesium. This tastes like chocolate but is very healthy – no guilt here!

Ingredients

4 tbsp coconut oil

4 tbsp organic 100% peanut butter or another nut spread

2 tsp raw honey or maple syrup

4 tbsp raw cacao powder

2 tsp maca or acai powder (optional
– use more cacao without)

A small handful of crushed nuts or seeds

Method

1. Heat a small saucepan slightly and add coconut oil, peanut butter and honey. You don't need it hot – just enough to melt the coconut oil and peanut butter until combined.

2. Mix in the cacao and maca/acai, then add the nuts/seeds.

3. Line a dish with baking paper, pour in the melted chocolate goodness and place in the freezer for five to ten minutes.

4. Take it out once solid and break up.

5. Store in a glass jar or container in the fridge or freezer.

What if you know what to eat, but still don't eat it?

What if you know what to eat to be healthy, but you still choose not to? Do you find that you just can't help yourself, even though you consciously should know better (well, at least after reading this book)? Emotional eating is something that most people can experience from time to time, including me. It can stem from a number of things, but the most common two are junk food's ability to make you feel temporarily better and a form of self-sabotage.

Biochemically speaking, when we eat foods that are high in fat and sugar they set off pleasure centres in the brain that tell you to eat more of them. In the caveman days, high carb and high fat meant a good source of energy, which is why your brain is wired to make you want to eat more of these foods. The other side of the coin is that junk foods are designed by corporations to have a 'bliss point' – a perfection in food chemistry that makes you want to eat more and more.

When we're stressed or emotional we often will try to fill a void by eating sugary foods that give us a temporary moment of pleasure. I know this feeling all too well – my brain is hardwired to want chocolate as soon as the shit hits the fan, so to speak (well, chocolate *and* wine actually). However, emotional eating isn't always annihilating a tub of ice cream in front of the TV. It can be the fact that you skip breakfast, don't bother preparing your meals or opt for unhealthy choices when you know they don't serve your body.

This emotional eating is frequently a form of self-sabotage – where you unknowingly consume things that you know will harm your body for underlying emotional reasons. In my experience, people who are truly happy and have the right tools available to them will usually make healthy choices. People who aren't happy, don't love themselves enough, and don't value themselves generally don't. One example is my mother, who is an emotional eater and always has been. She suffers from major depression and weighs over 120kg. Doctors are always telling her to exercise and eat well. The fact is, my mum knows exactly what to eat and what she needs to do to lose weight, but her lack of self-love and self-respect prevent her from loving herself enough to be healthy.

And my mum isn't alone – emotional eating nearly always comes from deep, subconscious beliefs. To discover your reasons behind why you do what you do, you must first start to really observe yourself and ask yourself honestly about why you are behaving in this way. A hypnotherapist, kinesiologist, energetic healer or another modality may be able to help with this (see Chapter 13).

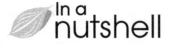

In a nutshell

There is no 'perfect' diet that suits everyone, so you need to listen to your body to figure out what works for you – focus on eating a varied diet, including carbohydrates, proteins and fats, to get a wide range of nutrients for your body to utilise.

Remember that eating healthily isn't about restriction – it's about eating wholesome, nutritious foods that will feed your body so it can function at its peak. When you decide to have a 'treat' make sure you enjoy it. You've been put on this Earth to live your life fully, so soak up the goodness of that occasional wine, chocolate or other treat guilt-free, knowing that the rest of your amazing diet allows you to do this without problems.

CHAPTER 8
DETOX – CLEAN UP YOUR ACT

'Cleansing is like my meditation. It makes me stop, focus and think about what I'm putting into my body. I'm making a commitment to my health and hitting the reset button.'
– SALMA HAYEK

Every single second of every day your cells are detoxifying. Unfortunately, even this regular detoxification isn't enough to deal with the swathe of toxins that we are exposed to on a day-to-day basis.

Think of your body as a garbage processing plant, with sorting chutes for paper, glass, food scraps and plastic. The garbage comes down conveyor belts at a steady rate to each of the chutes, which can only handle so much at once. Now imagine that the chute that takes the food scraps becomes blocked. The scraps begin to pile up as the new ones continue to come at a steady rate with nowhere to go. This is what it is like when one of your elimination organs blocks up – you end up with a big pile of garbage (toxins) that have nowhere to go, so have to accumulate in your body instead. We need to be able to help your body process the garbage and maintain the chutes to make sure they are flowing free.

So, how does it work?

Your body detoxifies through five main channels: the liver, kidneys, bowel, lymphatic system and skin.

Liver and bowel

Our livers really cop it. Your liver detoxifies almost everything in your body – from alcohol and chemicals to heavy metals and excess hormones and fats. Your liver has a big job, which is why I commonly see patients with a dysfunction of this important organ. If the liver is under prolonged stress, having to work hard to detoxify external toxins, it eventually starts to lose function. Once this happens, your ability to detoxify, digest and convert hormones in the body is impaired.

Liver and bowel detoxification are dependent on one another. The liver concentrates toxins in order to remove them from the body, which it largely does by the release of bile through the gall bladder. The gall bladder, which is an attachment of the liver, excretes bile into the duodenum (top of the small intestine) which then makes its way through the digestive tract, through the colon and is excreted in your bowel movements.

If you are constipated or your bowels are not moving regularly, then toxins released by the liver will have nowhere to go. A lot of the toxins that your liver processes every day will be reabsorbed by the body, so it is important that you keep the bowels moving well and have a good amount of fibre in your diet, which will assist the toxins in being removed from the body.

Your bowel flora is also very important for the detoxification and metabolism of excess hormones. Eating a diet rich in prebiotics like legumes, whole grains, fruit and veggies will help to foster healthy bowel flora.

Tips to love your liver

Start your day with the juice of a lemon in water – this stimulates bile flow and helps to activate your liver for the day.

Eat lots of green leafy veggies – your liver loves these. Avoid excessive alcohol intake, too much coffee and greasy foods – these put too much strain on your liver.

Drink lots of purified water. Eat bitter greens like watercress, rocket, dark lettuce leaves and dandelion greens. Eat fresh beetroot – not the canned variety.

Kidneys

Your kidneys detoxify you by filtering your blood. In fact, every hour your blood supply will pass though the kidneys twelve times and they'll process over 200 litres of blood a day! Filtration takes place in thousands of tiny tubules within the kidneys, which work hard to remove toxins and maintain the balance of minerals in your blood. Once the blood is cleaned it is returned into circulation.

Most people do not drink enough water. If you don't have enough water your blood volume will reduce, concentrating any toxins and putting more pressure on the kidneys. Our urine is an excellent way to remove toxins from the body and it should not be underestimated how vital drinking water is to this process.

Tips to love your kidneys

Drink at least 1.5 litres of water per day – more if you're exercising, drinking coffee or tea or in hot weather.

Eat lots of green leafy veggies (see a theme here?).

Enjoy fresh juices with celery – include the tops.

Drink lots of herbal tea – peppermint, chamomile, lemongrass, lemon, ginger.

Avoid excessive intake of coffee or tea (black, green or white), which puts a strain on the kidneys.

Lymphatic system

The lymphatic system is a network of lymphatic glands and vessels which collect fluid from the extremities and detoxify through lymphatic tissue. The lymphatic fluid is then put back into your blood circulation to be filtered by the kidneys.

The lymphatic system works by the pumping of fluid around the body by muscular movement. This means if you don't exercise regularly your lymphatic system cannot function properly. Skin congestion, cysts and boils are all signs of lymphatic congestion and the resultant toxicity.

Tips to love your lymphatic system

Drink lots of purified water. Exercise regularly – using your whole body, not just your legs. Have regular saunas or increase sweating with exercise. Dry skin brush every few days. Eat lots of green leafy veggies.

Dry skin brushing

Dry skin bruising is one of the easiest things you can do to stimulate your lymphatic system to cleanse your body. Here's how you do it:

1. *Before* showering, brush your skin with a natural bristle brush from your feet and hands towards your head in soft brisk strokes.
2. Rinse off in the shower. Do this every day while detoxing. While your skin should get a little bit red from this process, you should be gentle.

Skin

The largest organ in the body, your skin, actually works like a rudimentary kidney, releasing toxins by sweating. This makes exercise, steam rooms and saunas some great ways to detoxify through your skin.

If you find that you sweat too easily, soaking your clothes at the slightest bit of heat or movement, this is usually due to a dysfunction of the adrenal glands or kidneys.

Tips to love your skin

- Avoid the use of non-natural products on your skin.
- Never use aluminium-based deodorants or other intensive antiperspirants, which stop the production of sweat and allow these toxins to go straight into your bloodstream.

- Sweat regularly – exercise, sauna, steam rooms.
- Drink lots of water.
- Dry skin brush regularly.

Natural products

As well as releasing toxins from your body, your skin can also let toxins in.

To avoid this, use only 100 per cent natural skin care, hair care, styling products and make up. There are dozens of companies that offer excellent alternatives to their conventional counterparts. If you can't afford a full cupboard clean out, start with things that are going to be left on your skin like moisturisers, make up and perfume.

The same goes for cleaning products, which don't only make contact with the skin but can also be inhaled. Look for natural alternatives to cleaning products, especially the ones you use every day like dishwashing liquid or tablets, laundry detergents and surface sprays. Never use air fresheners or fly spray, which are an easy way to distribute chemicals around your home.

Emotions and the organs

In Traditional Chinese Medicine each organ has an emotion associated with it. These emotions can affect your organs, and dysfunction in your organs can cause emotional difficulties. In my practice I have found that when I mention these emotions to patients they are often met by a realisation. Emotional connections to illness are very common, contributing to and exacerbating health issues.

Liver
The emotions associated with the liver are anger and frustration. Being snappy or easily annoyed can be a sign that your liver is unhappy.

Kidneys
The kidneys are associated with fear, worry and concern. Anxiety can be linked to the kidneys and fear of a negative outcome.

Bowels
Grief and sadness are associated with the bowel. Constipation can mean that we're holding on to old emotions.

How to spring clean your body

Now that you know how your amazing body naturally detoxifies your cells, you're ready to explore the different ways that you can help your body do its job. Regular detoxification will help reduce fatigue, improve sleep, balance hormones, improve digestion and even prevent ageing.

Thankfully there are many methods of detoxification that work so you don't have to stick to one type. The principle of any detoxification program is to give your body a break from daily toxins and to give it a helping hand in the detoxification process. In this section you'll learn some basic methods of detoxification and how they might help. In the *Resources* section I'll also go into more detail with detox plans for the novice, intermediate and advanced detoxer.

Elimination detox
The type of detox I recommend most frequently is an elimination detox. This style of detox removes common toxins from the diet, replacing them with foods that help to heal and detoxify the body. In a perfect world, this type of diet would be what we consumed

all day every day, but in reality it is not sustainable or completely necessary for most people.

During an elimination diet, I advise the removal of the following foods:

- Sugar – and anything with added sugar
- Dairy (milk, cheese) – except a little probiotic yoghurt (unless you're dairy sensitive)
- Gluten (you can try just wheat free if eliminating gluten is too difficult)
- Processed food – anything premade or pre-packaged
- Coffee and black tea
- Alcohol

For some, this list will seem overwhelming. However, eliminating all of these food groups will give your body the best chance to detoxify and heal, and will give it a break from digesting wheat and dairy, which take a lot of energy to break down. This energy can be better spent by the body on the process of detoxification.

Substitutions

But what will I eat? It's a question that I get all the time. Here are some handy substitutions that will help you to clean up your act.

- **Milk** – Use rice milk, oat milk or almond milk instead (see page 135 for recipe). Luckily you won't be drinking coffee so no need to worry about milk there!

- **Cheese** – Cheese is a food with a high level of attachment and is often the hardest to give up. Try replacing cheese with olives or olive tapenades, dips or avocado to give your meals that little something extra that you may be missing.

- **Bread** – Bread is difficult, and you won't really find a gluten-free alternative that is not processed as many commercial gluten-free breads are full of additives and chemicals to get them to taste like normal bread. If you're going wheat-free, then spelt or khorasan bread are good alternatives – sourdough is best.
- **Coffee** – My best advice here is to just give it up if you can. You could also try roasted dandelion root tea (brewed in your coffee machine).
- **Black tea** – Try switching to green tea or rooibos, an African tea that tastes like tea (well sort of) without the tannins or caffeine.
- **Sugar** – Try using honey, xylitol or maple syrup, if you need to (see Chapter 7 for more info).

I usually recommend people do this type of detox at least once per year to help clean the body and allow for healing. The best way to do this is coupled with a course of herbal and nutritional detox agents that will help support your organs of elimination through the process. It's worthwhile checking in with your naturopath for this, who will not only give you powerful and tailored medicines to help get the most out of the detox, but can identify which organs need the most help and what type of detox will suit you best.

Chia seeds for detoxification

Chia seeds are an excellent addition for detox due to the high levels of mucilage and soluble fibre. This fibre helps pull toxins out of the gut and acts as a prebiotic to help give your good bacteria some food to munch on. For best results, pre-soak 2 tbsp of chia seeds in water then eat it each day of detoxing. You can put it in a smoothie, in yoghurt or into porridge or muesli.

Juicing for detoxification

Fresh juicing is an excellent method for detoxing. You can juice as a part of any detox program, or can undertake a juice fast where you drink only juice to give your body a chance to heal.

Fresh juices work well because by taking away the fibre you are left with a concentrated source of nutrition and phytonutrients that will help your body detoxify.

I don't recommend that you undertake a juice fast while you are under the day-to-day stress of working, studying or other activities that may tax your energy. Drinking only juices can cause strong detox reactions which, although beneficial, are not convenient in a working environment. To get the most out of any type of fast you need to be in a supportive environment where you are able to nurture yourself and reflect on your feelings as it can be quite an emotional process.

One thing that I do recommend is a weekend juice fast – where you may drink only freshly made juice from Friday evening to Monday morning. You can then use this as part of your detox program to help give your body a boost of nutrition and allow it to go into the detoxification process more deeply.

Properties of fresh juices

Each fruit and veggie will have different effects so I recommend getting a variety in to get a broad range of benefits.

- Apple juice contains quercetin, a bioflavonoid which is anti-allergic, anti-inflammatory and immune modulating. It *is* present in the skin, though, so a cold-pressed juicer is best to extract this nutrient.
- Beetroot juice is particularly good for your liver and cardiovascular system. It helps to cleanse blood and is packed with antioxidants.
- Broccoli-stem juice is a great way to use up your stems. It has anticancer properties and can help to balance hormones. It is also a source of vitamin C.
- Carrot juice is excellent for improving eyesight, being

high in vitamin A.

- Celery juice is the best for kidney cleansing. It also contains compounds which are thought to be anti-ageing. Make sure you juice the tops, which have concentrated nutrients.
- Cucumber juice is very cleansing and can help to heal your cells. Drink it for glowing skin.
- Garlic juice is antibacterial, antiviral and anti-inflammatory. It's also great for heart health and your immune system.
- Ginger juice helps to boost circulation and is a potent anti-inflammatory. It's best to have ginger with your juice in colder months or if you are a 'cold' person.
- Kale juice is the ultimate super food – it helps to detoxify excess hormones and cleanse your body. It's also a great source of iron, calcium and magnesium.
- Lemon juice is extremely alkalising (anti-inflammatory) in the body. It also helps to stimulate liver function and is a source of vitamin C.
- Pineapple juice is a rich source of vitamin C and the bioflavonoid bromelain, a phytonutrient which has been found to be anti-cancer, anti-inflammatory and anti-allergic. Bromelain is especially concentrated in the core.
- Spinach juice is high in blood-cleansing chlorophyll, iron, calcium and magnesium. It's also an excellent source of folate.
- Watermelon juice contains the amino acid citrulline, which is needed for cardiovascular health. It is also high in lycopene, another nutrient that benefits heart health.
- Wheat grass juice is a powerhouse of vitamins and minerals. It is one of the highest sources of chlorophyll, which helps to oxygenate the blood and detoxify the body.

TIP: *Juicing sprouts, herbs like parsley and basil, and super greens like dandelion will really give you a super boost of nutrients that will kick your body into healing mode.*

Fasting

Fasting is something that I discovered several years ago when I visited a wonderful retreat called Natural Instinct Healing in Bali. Here I undertook a ten-day fast and never turned back! If I have the time available, this is something that I try to do every year as a powerful method of detoxification. As with straight juice fasting, I do not recommend fasting as an activity that you undertake as part of your day-to-day life. Going to a specialised retreat ensures that you will be looked after during the process and have the important 'you time' that you'll need to get the most out of the process.

Fasting has been used since the beginning of time to prevent ageing and detoxify the mind and body. Fasting should always be accompanied by a colon-cleansing program involving colonics or enemas to help to drag toxins out of the bowel. Fasting in conjunction with enemas or colonics is the only way to remove plaque from the bowel, which builds up over the years and impairs our health.

Taking food away from the body allows the energy that normally goes into digestion to go towards healing your tissues and organs and you are able to see some powerful changes occur. It can also allow suppressed emotions to come to the surface, allowing you to really deal with issues that may be holding you back from living your life fully. It's not for the faint hearted, but I do recommend that you try it if you want to reach optimum health.

Intermittent fasting for health

There is some good evidence that intermittent fasting or intermittent calorie restriction can be beneficial for your health. In some methods, it is recommended that for two days per week you eat only one small meal. This can help to give your body a bit of a break which allows healing. During these 'fasting' days it is important that you keep hydrated with water, herbal teas and coconut water. You can have some watered down freshly made juice as well if desired. This doesn't work for everyone so give it a try and see how your body responds.

Choosing the right detox for you

Any amount of cleansing is going to be more beneficial to your body than none at all. You need to decide which type of detox will be best for your body. If you're new to this crazy world of detoxing than perhaps try a shorter timeframe and work your way up to longer periods of elimination. In the *Resources* section, you can find detox plans for the novice (ten days), intermediate (twenty-one days) and advanced (more than thirty days) – do whatever is most comfortable for you so you can get the best results.

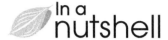

In a nutshell

Detoxification is essential for every single one of us. It helps to rid your body of toxins, clean up your diet and give your body the nutrition that it needs to heal without the burden of processing detrimental foods, alcohol or coffee.

While your body is naturally designed to detox, by choosing to go on a detox plan you can help it recover from the stressors and toxins of your everyday environment. For more information on the detoxes in this chapter, refer to the easy detox plans in the Resources section.

CHAPTER 9
RELAX – ZEN YOUR
WAY TO HEALTH

*'When you get into your car, shut the door and be there
for just half a minute. Breathe, feel the energy inside
your body, look around at the sky, the trees. The mind
might tell you, 'I don't have time.' But that's the mind
talking to you. Even the busiest person has time for
thirty seconds of space.'*
– ECKHART TOLLE

In this busy world we rarely take the time that we need to wind down. We push the limits with late bedtimes and early wakeups; ignoring our bodies' need for sleep. We get so caught up in the busyness of our lives that we neglect our bodies' cries for rest and relaxation. However, with the lifestyle, environmental and dietary stressors of everyday life, this rest is essential for healing.

So where do you start? Fortunately there are a number of ways you can integrate relaxation into your everyday life, along with plenty of ways you can improve your sleep.

Relaxation as a health tool

More than 3,000 studies have shown benefits in the effect of relaxation on a wide range of conditions, including anxiety, asthma, depression, diabetes, fibromyalgia, headaches, heart disease, high blood pressure, hot flushes, insomnia, irritable bowel syndrome, nightmares, overactive bladder, pain, PMS, smoking cessation, temporomandibular joint (TMJ) pain and tension headaches.

Why does it work?
From Chapter 5 you know that stress triggers your fight or flight response. This results in your adrenal glands pumping out cortisol, and your energy and blood being diverted from the 'non-essential' digestive and reproductive systems to be pumped into your muscles and brain. The ultimate result is that stress disrupts the way that your digestive, detoxifying and reproductive organs work, and the longer you are in a state of stress, the greater the imbalance.

Relaxation techniques like meditation, guided visualisation, self-hypnosis, and deep breathing reduce this stress response, which allows your body to come back to homeostasis more easily and focus on healing.

How can you do it?
Relaxation is an individual thing, which means you may need to try several methods to see what works for you. Some of the most common types of relaxation include breathing techniques, meditation, conscious body relaxation and self-hypnosis.

Technique 1 – Breathing
The easiest thing you can do to help reduce cortisol and alleviate stress is to breathe properly. In fact, a study published in the journal Chest in 2000 indicated that how well the lungs take in and release air was a predictor of mortality in the general population. In the study, which assessed over 1000 individuals, it was found that the less air that was expired through the lungs, the higher the chance that people would die sooner. It stands to reason that if we exercise our lungs like we do the rest of our bodies, then we have a much better chance of living a long and healthy life.

However, most people aren't experiencing the benefits of deep breathing because they only breathe with the top third of their lungs. This shallow breathing causes even more stress and tension in the body, as well as depriving you of oxygen, which will affect your energy levels. If we are to truly gain the amazing health benefits that our lungs afford us then we must break the habit of poor breathing and use our lungs properly.

Breathing using your whole lungs

1. Visualise your lungs coming all the way down into your belly (which they pretty much do).

2. Exhale.

3. Breathing in, imagine that you are filling your lungs with air from the bottom up, like you are filling a glass with water. Continue breathing in until you have filled your lungs with air from the base right up to the top (just under your collarbones).

4. Exhale slowly, releasing the air from the top of the lungs first, and then emptying the lungs right down into the belly. Imagine the level of water in the glass dropping.

5. Use this visualisation to help you get a feel for how to use your whole lungs.

It will take a number of weeks or even months to retrain your breathing habits. Stress inherently impairs our respiration – it is a natural instinct to hold our breath when in a flight and fight state so you need to consciously monitor your breathing to keep it in check. If you find yourself feeling stressed, take several slow, deep breaths to calm your body. This is the most effective way to reduce tension on the spot – you take your lungs everywhere you go and it's free.

Breathing exercises to calm your body

There are many breathing exercises out there that help to calm your body. I have listed three easy ones that you can integrate into your day. Try each of them and see what works best for you.

Coherent breathing

This simple method is based on the theory that when you breathe slowly and coherently it balances the autonomic nervous system. Your autonomic nervous system controls all of the 'automatic' functions in the body, like your digestion, breathing and heartbeat.

To practice coherent breathing, you need to take five breaths per minute. This is a simple as breathing in for five counts and breathing out for five counts. To help keep your counts slow and consistent try counting using 'Mississippi' (as in, 'one-Mississippi, two Mississippi,' and so on). You don't need to force the breath – just let it flow gently in and out.

Try this practice lying down with your eyes closed for ten minutes a day and see how you feel. There are many MP3s and smartphone apps that have been created to help you time your breath correctly.

1. Lie or sit in a comfortable position.
2. Exhale. Take a slow deep breath in to the count of five.
3. Exhale slowly to the count of five, without force.
4. Repeat.

Breath moving

Breath moving involves visualising your breath moving through different parts of your body. This can help give your mind something to focus on during the relaxation process, which is helpful if you can't still your mind.

1. Get in a comfortable position, either sitting or lying.
2. As you breathe in slowly, visualise your breath moving to the top of your head.

3. As you breathe out slowly, visualise the breath moving to the base of your spine, through your pelvis, your sit bones and your perineum.
4. Each time you breathe in, visualise the breath moving back to the top of the head.
5. Each time you breathe out; move the breath back down the spine and into the pelvis and sit bones again.
6. Repeat this at least ten times.

Alternate nostril breathing

Alternate nostril breathing, traditionally known as nadi shohan pranayama, is a yogic breathing technique that helps to calm the mind and energise the body. Even a few minutes a day of alternate nostril breathing will help to de-stress your mind and relieve tension.

Alternate nostril breathing involves rhythmically breathing through just one of your nostrils at a time. By alternating sides it is thought to connect the left (logical) and right (emotional) hemispheres of the brain, helping them to integrate and provide balance in moods and emotional wellbeing.

1. Sit in a comfortable position with your spine straight and your shoulders relaxed. Place your left hand on your knee.
2. Rest the tips of your right middle and index fingers on your brow line, in between the eyes. Place your ring finger and the thumb on the sides of the nose. You will use these fingers to block your nostrils.
3. Press your thumb over the right nostril.
4. Exhale through the left nostril, then inhale through the left nostril.
5. Take your thumb off the right nostril and block the left nostril with your ring finger.
6. Exhale through the right nostril, then inhale through the same nostril.

7. Switch to the other side.

8. Continue to inhale then exhale from alternate nostrils.

Try this for a few minutes and see how you feel. Remember to breathe gently but deeply, always inhaling from the same nostril after exhaling.

With any breathing technique, the key is consistency. Try a technique for a few minutes twice per day for two weeks and see how you feel. A great time for this is on rising and before bed, or perhaps at intervals during your work day to help to de-stress.

Technique 2 – Meditation

Meditation is another form of relaxation, and has been used by cultures all over the world to create inner peace and improve wellbeing. There are hundreds of studies on the effects of meditation on health, with most showing positive outcomes. Notably, a 2012 review of 163 studies that examined transcendental meditation found that it had marked effects in reducing anxiety, negative emotions and neuroticism, while improving learning, memory and self-realisation.

Meditation is particularly useful for reducing stress and improving mood issues like anxiety and depression. It helps you to focus on the present and regular practice can help keep you in tune with your body.

Types of meditation

There are many types of meditation and variants of these types. Some examples are zazen or seated meditation, where there is no focus, mantra meditation where you meditate using chanting or voice, guided visualisations, and kundalini meditation, where you focus on your energy centres (chakras).

I have found guided visualisation and mantra meditation to be the easiest way to get started.

Visualisation

Guided meditation or visualisation is a good place
to start, as all you need to do is find a comfortable
place and listen to a CD or an MP3. You can even get
meditation apps on your phone, which you can listen
to whenever you have a free ten to fifteen minutes. In
these audio tracks you'll be guided to imagine different
images or thoughts, which help to break you out of any
negative patterns that could be causing tension.

There are many different styles of guided meditation
– if you don't like the first one you try, then keep looking
for different ones. You can get guided meditations based
on relaxing your muscles, clearing your chakras, healing
with angels and even ones that are more religious-based
if you wish. I enjoy listening to guided meditations by the
intuitive healer Kate Reardon (katereardon.com.au) and
Doreen Virtue (angeltherapy.com).

You can also guide yourself through a visualisation
without audio cues. Something simple like the
visualisation below is a good place to start – all you
need to do is use your imagination.

1. Lie down in a comfortable position. You may like to put
   on some gentle music or sit outside and listen to the
   sounds of nature.
2. Take several deep breaths, using one of the techniques
   on pages 170-172.
3. Imagine that you are walking on the beach. The sand
   is warm underneath your bare feet. Hear the waves softly
   breaking on the shore and feel the soft, salty breeze in your hair.
4. You look out to the beach. The water is crystal clear with
   pure white sand beneath. There is no one else on the
   beach – you have it all to yourself.
5. Slowly you walk towards the water's edge. As you dip
   your feet into the water you find that it is the perfect
   temperature. You feel safe and secure.

6. You walk into the water and feel its soft caress against your body. Once you're in up to your waist you lie down and float in the water.

7. As you float on your back you feel weightless. You can feel the warm sun on the front of your body and it seems to energise you.

8. Bring your awareness to any negative thoughts or feelings you have. Focus on any worry, pain or discomfort. Once you have these feelings let them drift from your body into the cleansing water.

9. Imagine the water washing away any fears or concerns you have. Exchange them for the pure, invigorating energy from the warm sun on your skin.

10. Sit in this place for as long as you'd like, then, once you are ready, get out of the water, take several deep breaths and come back into the present.

Visualisation is a very powerful method of relaxation and healing. We'll talk more about the power of visualisation in Chapter 12.

Mantra meditation

Mantra meditation involves repeating mantras over and over in a rhythmic fashion to incite relaxation. Mantra is a Sanskrit word meaning sacred utterance, or numinous sound – you can use a word, syllable or group of words. According to Deepak Chopra, a mantra is an instrument of the mind, a powerful sound or vibration that you can use to enter a deeper state of meditation. Mantra meditation can be done on your own, with music or even by chanting along to an MP3 or app. You don't have to say mantras out loud; they can be repeated in your mind quietly to help take the focus off busy thoughts so you can focus on the practice of meditation.

Some ancient mantras include:

- Om (or Aum) – The most well known mantra, this is considered to be the most elemental sound, representing infinite universal consciousness.

- Om Namah Shivaya – translated to 'I honour the divinity within myself', this mantra can help with self-love and confidence.

You could also use single words:
- Shradda – Faith
- Bhakti – Devotion
- Shanti – Peace
- Prajna – Wisdom
- Ananda – Bliss

I'd recommend getting some MP3s, apps or even searching for some of these mantras on YouTube to hear how they sound and to get used to saying them.

Modern-day mantras

A mantra for you can also be a positive phrase that you say over and over to help to relax you or heal your mind. Good examples are:
- 'I am ... healthy, loved, happy, energised' or whatever positive words you'd like to use. You can also simply say 'I am', which has powerful connotations itself.
- 'Today I choose ... joy, love, happiness, peace' – whatever you would like to choose today.
- 'Every day in every way, I am getting better and better' – a positive quote by Laura Silva.
- 'I change my thoughts, I change my world' – this quote by Norman Vincent Peale is a good reminder.
- 'This too, shall pass' – good for when you are stuck in a very negative mindset or can't overcome a challenge.

Once you have some practice with mantra or guided meditation, you may find that you can clear your mind and just be still with your thoughts. Most people think that if you can't do this you can't meditate, but this certainly isn't the case. The aim of meditation is to calm your mind and allow for inner stillness and self-reflection. If you are unable to create a stillness in your mind without the aid of mantras or visualisations it doesn't matter – these tools will still give you the same effect. In other words, you don't need to be a Buddhist monk to reap the benefits of meditation!

Technique 3 – Conscious body relaxation

The next technique is simply using your mind to relax your body, which in turn will help you to move into a deeper state of mental relaxation. There is a great audio track created by Kate Reardon which is designed to help you do this, and works particularly well if you feel really tense or have a lot of mental chatter (as in your mind just won't shut up!). It's called 'healing the body meditation' - you can find it at katereardon.com/store.

You can also try this simple exercise at home:

1. Lie in a comfortable position. Play some gentle music if desired, or listen to the sounds of nature.
2. Take several deep breaths, using the techniques on pages 170-172.
3. With each exhalation, focus on relaxing one area of your body. You can start with your toes, your feet, your left leg, then right leg, your butt, your hips, your internal organs, your left arm, then your right arm, your chest, your lower back, your upper back, your neck, your head, your face, your lips, your eyes and your jaw.
4. Each time you breathe out, relax the area of focus and feel it get heavy, sinking into the floor.
5. Once you have done your whole body take several deep breaths and feel your whole body relaxing, feeling heavy and sinking into the floor.

Technique 4 – Self-hypnosis

The last relaxation technique I'd like to share with you is self-hypnosis. Self-hypnosis is a form of stress reduction therapy that helps you to reach a deeper level of relaxation. Like guided meditation, there are many MP3s and apps available to download that are designed to bring you into a state of hypnosis. When you are in this trance-like state, you can access your subconscious mind and release tension and fears on a deeper level.

In a self-hypnosis track, you'll be given cues to help you go deeper and deeper into relaxation. When this is working well, you'll feel your body getting heavier and heavier and it is a fantastic feeling to be so relaxed.

Self-hypnosis is great for stress relief, confidence and self-esteem issues, sleep problems and anxiety. You can also get audio tracks for these specific areas of concern, as well as more general ones.

Sleep away your symptoms

Beyond using relaxation techniques throughout your day-to-day routine, getting plenty of sleep is essential to your health and healing.

Sleep does sooo much more for us than recharging our batteries. When I first learnt about what happens while we sleep, I was amazed. During this seemingly inert part of your day (or night, rather), your body is repairing damage, detoxifying, balancing your hormones and even processing your memories. Without enough good-quality sleep your body cannot heal or repair. Lack of sleep has also been linked to weight gain, anxiety, depression and many diseases.

So here's the way it works. During the night, your body undergoes a sleep cycle – a complex event which starts with falling asleep, then changes in intensity and function throughout the night until you wake up in the morning.

When we sleep there are two main cycles – REM (rapid eye movement) sleep and non-REM sleep. In the first part of the night, ideally from 9pm to 1am, our sleep is predominantly non-REM.

During non-REM sleep, the body is completing all of its most vital functions – healing and repairing, detoxifying, hormone balancing and cellular regeneration (anti-ageing).

After the first part of the night, you will transition into bigger and bigger portions of REM sleep until you wake. During REM sleep we are balancing moods and processing all of the information that we took in the previous day. Part of REM sleep involves dreaming, which is why we remember our dreams when we wake up in the morning, because we are dreaming just prior to waking.

Our sleep is so vital to our health that it is the first thing that I look to correct with my patients. The effect of sleep on healing cannot be underestimated, so it's important that you make sure you're getting enough.

How do I know if I'm getting enough sleep?

We need a minimum of eight hours of sleep a night to properly heal and repair the body. With our busy lives, there are a lot of people who simply are not getting enough, believing that they need just enough to get by, rather than making it an essential part of their lifestyle. Studies show that anything less than seven hours of sleep a night puts you at serious risk of developing disease. Although some people can get by on seven hours, in my experience I find that most of us need at least eight hours to really get what we need. Perhaps this would be different if our bodies did not have to deal with the huge amount of toxins that we are exposed to every day.

The time of sleep is also important. Studies have found that most of our 'repairing' sleep – where we regenerate and detoxify – happens between 9pm and 1am. This means if you're hitting the hay at the 10pm or 11pm mark, or later, you'll be missing out on your most important sleep of the night.

The sleep initiation process is also important. You should be able to fall asleep easily, without any aid, within five to ten minutes. Anything more than this means that your sleep cycle is not being initiated properly due to stress, hormonal or neurotransmitter imbalances or issues with your sleep cycle. 'Passing out' is also a sign that you have problems with your sleep. Usually from exhaustion, immediately passing out does not give your body time to initiate the sleep cycle properly and can lead to poor sleep quality.

Besides turning over every now and then, you should sleep right through the night. If you do wake briefly, you should barely notice and easily drift right back into a deep sleep.

If you aren't getting enough sleep, or your sleep-wake cycle isn't working for you, you'll probably notice some of the following:

- It takes longer than ten minutes to fall asleep.
- You are a very light sleeper, being woken up with even the slightest disturbance.
- You wake up during the night.
- You don't remember your dreams.
- You wake up feeling tired and groggy or wanting to stay in bed and sleep some more.
- You're not getting enough sleep, due to going to bed too late, waking up early, taking ages to fall asleep or waking during the night.

Dreamtime

Do you remember your dreams? It's a question that I ask my patients every visit. If you don't remember your dreams when you wake up it can mean that you're not getting enough quality sleep to switch into longer periods of REM sleep in the early hours. You don't need to remember details or remember them for long, but you should have an awareness that you have been dreaming. When I work on correcting adrenal function and supporting my clients' nervous systems, they soon begin to dream again which tells me that their sleep cycles are correcting.

How do you feel when you wake up in the morning? Do you feel rested and refreshed? If the answer is no then you are not getting enough sleep, or your sleep quality needs work. Some people report sleeping for twelve hours and still feeling terrible. This usually means that your sleep cycles are not doing what they are meant to and you're missing out on restorative sleep. This can often be an issue for shift workers and night owls who miss their restorative sleep.

The ideal sleep

In the ideal sleep you'd go to bed at 9pm and wake up at 5am to get the full healing effect between 9pm and 1am. You'd sleep for a minimum of eight hours. This is from the time you are actually asleep – not when you go to bed. You'll fall asleep within five to ten minutes. You'll sleep all the way through the night. You may move or turn occasionally but you should barely remember doing so. You wake up feeling rested and refreshed – like you have had a good night's sleep. You'll also remember your dreams, at least for a moment when you rise.

Perfect sleep

Go to bed at 9pm.

Take five to ten minutes to fall asleep.

Sleep all the way through the night.

Wake at 5am feeling refreshed and rested.

Remember your dreams.

Anything outside this sleep picture is not ideal and will not give you the full health benefits that you need from sleep.

What's causing my sleep problems?

The two main sleeping problems people experience are difficulty falling asleep, and difficulty staying asleep.

Difficulty falling asleep, or sleep onset insomnia, can be due to high levels of cortisol. Cortisol is your 'awake' hormone, and should be nice and high during the morning and lunchtime and begin to drop off in the afternoon. This drop in cortisol signals the beginning of the sleep cycle to your body, so if cortisol remains elevated because of stress then this can leave you wide awake when you're trying to fall asleep.

Another cause of sleep onset problems is neurotransmitter (your mood hormones) deficiencies. A lack of serotonin, for example, will lead to a reduction in the production of your sleep hormone melatonin, as it is what melatonin is made from. If you lack the nutrients to convert serotonin into melatonin, such as zinc, magnesium and B6, you're also in trouble because your body won't be able to make enough melatonin to initiate sleep.

The other issue is an overstimulation of the sympathetic nervous system – or your flight and fight response. Sleep requires relaxation and if your body can't relax because of stress, nervous tension or emotional issues, then it will impair your ability to fall asleep.

If you fall asleep but can't stay asleep, then you could also have abnormal cortisol levels during the night, or a deficiency of melatonin. Improving adrenal health usually fixes sleep maintenance issues. You may also need to look at when you wake up during the night – according to the Chinese body clock, waking between 1am and 3am means that your liver is unhappy, and in my clinical experience, I find this to be very accurate. Often when we work on improving liver function, the 2am wake ups stop.

So how can you sleep like a baby?

The difficulty with improving your sleep is that once it is out of whack it causes fatigue and adrenal exhaustion, which in turn lead to more sleep problems and so on and so forth. You may need to see a natural health professional to help with your nervous system and adrenals in order to get things corrected if your sleep is chronically bad. For milder cases, though, improving your sleep hygiene may help.

Sleep hygiene is the process of priming your body for bedtime. Think dark room, comfortable bed and quiet time. Here are some great tips to help with regulating your sleep/ wake cycle:

1. Increase energy throughout the day

You need adequate energy levels to initiate sleep and help with sleep processes. A naturopath can prescribe you herbal medicines and nutritional supplements to support energy production, but a lot can be done through the diet too. Aim for complex carbohydrates, lots of fresh fruit and vegetables and limit your sugar intake.

2. Avoid stimulants later in the day

Try to avoid having any coffee, soft drink, black or green tea or dark chocolate after 2pm. Those who are sensitive to the effects of caffeine should try to avoid these things altogether.

3. Avoid starches at night

Starches are difficult to break down and can disrupt the sleep process. Avoid having any potato, white rice, pasta, bread or noodles with dinner. Complex carbohydrates like brown rice or quinoa are fine.

4. Sleep in a dark room

Complete darkness helps to promote good levels of sleep-regulating melatonin. Waking up to a bright light also helps to promote a good sleep cycle, so turn on the light or open the curtains when you wake up.

5. Exercise on rising

Doing some star jumps or balancing exercises on rising has been shown to help regulate the sleep/wake cycle – the movement tells your body you are awake. Even sixty seconds will help.

6. No screen time before bed

Try not to look at any screens at least forty-five minutes before bed. Studies show that the light from the screen stimulates your pituitary gland and makes it difficult for your body to start the sleep cycle. This means no playing candy crush or checking emails on your phone in bed!

7. Promote a state of calm around bedtime

Try to set a routine to wind down at night, avoiding TV and computer use before bed (as mentioned above). Try putting some lavender oil on your pillow and doing some deep breathing exercises before bed to instil a state of calm. You can read a book, but you might want to avoid books that are too exciting or stimulating (*Game of Thrones* may not be the best choice).

8. Get a comfortable, well-supported bed and pillows

You spend around one-third of your life in bed so it's worthwhile investing in a quality mattress. Pillows that support your neck properly will help prevent neck pain or discomfort. If your body is uncomfortable or painful, then consider seeing a chiropractor, osteopath or massage therapist to help.

Remember, the sleep cycle actually starts hours before bed with your body reducing cortisol, which it uses to keep you awake and alert, and increasing melatonin even before you sleep. If falling asleep is an issue for you, try to have a relaxing and calm evening free from stress and over stimulation.

Times when you'll need more sleep

There are times in your life where your body will need more sleep than usual. These are:

- During illnesses like colds, flus and viruses;
- If healing from major injuries like burns, breaks and fractures;
- During pregnancy;
- During birth recovery and breastfeeding (good luck with that one!);
- During times of high stress (yes, like the times when you're up super late because you're so busy at work); and
- During detoxification.

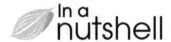

In a nutshell

Adequate rest and relaxation is an essential part of our healing journey. Our body needs good-quality sleep to be able to repair damage, detoxify, balance hormones and process memories. Additionally, learning to integrate relaxation techniques such as breathing exercises or meditation into your day-to-day routine will help you reduce stress, so your body can focus on staying in balance, rather than getting stuck in fight or flight mode.

CHAPTER 10
EXERCISE (DO I REALLY HAVE TO?)

'A healthy body means a healthy mind. You get your heart rate up, and you get the blood flowing through your body to your brain. Look at Albert Einstein. He rode a bicycle. He was also an early student of Jazzercise. You never saw Einstein lift his shirt, but he had a six-pack under there.'

— STEVE CARELL

If you're eating properly, detoxing and getting enough sleep, do you really need to exercise? Yes, you do. Why?

Because our bodies are designed to move. They aren't designed to sit at a desk for eight hours a day, followed by an hour in the car and then four hours in front of the TV. They function best when we give them regular movement.

To maintain a healthy body weight, exercise is essential. And this is just as important whether or not you're overweight, as without exercise our organs can become coated in visceral fat, even if we look 'skinny' on the outside. This fat is more dangerous to our health than the stuff we can see, which means that skinny people aren't necessarily healthy people.

It's not all about weight loss, though. When we exercise it changes our biochemistry – every cell in the body is affected in a positive way. Studies have found that exercise is linked to reduced insulin resistance, increases in feel-good endorphins, a reduction in inflammatory markers, decreases in blood pressure and changes in neurotransmitters (your mood-regulating hormones).

Exercising can also change your eating habits. A study published in the American Journal of Clinical Nutrition found that when people became more active they were more satisfied with the same amount of food, suggesting that exercise makes us more in tune with our bodies' hunger signals. I have observed this in my practice, as well as the effect of regular exercise making people choose healthier food options.

What else can exercise do?

- Move blood around the body, ensuring the nutrients it contains can get where they are needed;
- Help you metabolise fat and build muscle;
- Help you detoxify by pulling toxins from your extremities;
- Reduce insulin resistance (prevents diabetes);
- Increase your energy;
- Improve your sleep;
- Improve mood;
- Improve your sex life; and
- Help manage your stress by increasing your feel-good hormones (endorphins) and balancing your energy levels.

This is why if you're not exercising regularly, it's time to get started.

How much is enough?

The Mayo Clinic recommends that you get 150 minutes of moderate aerobic activity (like brisk walking, swimming, mowing the lawn or low intensity cycling) or seventy-five minutes of vigorous activity (running, aerobics, gym classes or dancing) a week. That equates to around three fifty-minute sessions per week if moderate, or three twenty-five-minute intensive sessions.

Strength training is also important, such as weights or weight-bearing activities like strengthening yoga poses, Pilates, squats, lunges and push ups. There is no recommended amount of time for these sessions; however I would aim for at least twenty minutes a week here.

More than this is great, but there is a limit. Unless you are training for a marathon or are an elite athlete you don't want to be doing intensive exercise more than five days a week. Walking, jogging, yoga and Pilates are, however, excellent daily practices.

That said, like relaxation, exercise is also an individual thing and some people need more than others to feel good.

So think about what you like, and what will fit in to your life. Do you enjoy the calmer pace of a yoga class, or do you feel great after a higher intensity run? Do you feel better doing twenty minutes of exercise every day, or do you prefer doing two one-hour sessions a week?

If you aren't sure, try it out – most gyms and classes offer trials if you want to do something structured, or if you want to get into nature all you need are your running shoes. It's important to note that it takes around two weeks to get used to a new exercise routine, to see if it makes you feel good or not. So set yourself a commitment – can you stick to a new program, struggle through it for just two weeks? You'll be pleasantly surprised at the results if you do.

Which type of exercise is best?

There is no one exercise that is suitable for every single person. Likewise, there is no clear-cut answer on if there is more benefit in doing intensive or gentle exercise, as it depends on your body type and the state of your health.

As a general rule, it is good to have a blend of aerobic exercise (stuff that gets your heart pumping), strength work, and weight-bearing exercise (this puts pressure on our bones, making them stronger and preventing osteoporosis, and includes walking, running, cycling, weights and most sports).

Generally for weight loss, diabetes control and cardiovascular health, intensive exercise will work best as it burns more calories, gets your heart rate higher and works up more of a sweat.

Gentle exercise, on the other hand, has the benefit of helping you to de-stress and unwind, giving you time to mentally process thoughts. Certain types of gentle exercise, such as yoga, can be very toning and improve your flexibility. Yoga is one of my favourite forms of exercise – not only does it help with fitness, toning and flexibility, it has a holistic element that looks at breathing and meditation as part of the practice, which really rounds out the benefits. Some yoga poses can compress parts of the body like joints and organs, which helps to create a rebound flow of blood to the site. Blood carries all of your oxygen, nutrients and chemical mediators around the body, and yoga can help target specific areas to enhance their function.

It is good to have a blend of high intensity and low intensity exercise in your routine if you can, which will afford you the benefits of both. That said, the most important thing is finding something that you like doing enough so that you will keep doing it!

For more information about different types of exercise and the pros and cons of each, look at Exercise resources in the Resources section.

Cleaning and gardening

Beyond going out of your way to exercise, did you know you can get fit while gardening or cleaning the toilet? This incidental exercise will add to your overall fitness, so put some elbow grease into it! Gardening also gives you the added benefit of being out in nature, which is a win-win for your health, as you'll discover next chapter.

Activity	Kj[1] burned per half hour
Ironing	260
Making the bed	290
Vacuuming	370
Gardening	630
Mowing the lawn	840
Hanging out the washing	504

Source: Fitness Australia

---

1   Kilojoules are a way of measuring the energy in food. If you prefer calories, just divide by 4.2.

Stretching

Stretching in its simplest form is a natural and instinctive activity that all animals, including humans, do regularly. Instinctively it feels good to stretch – your body knows that stretching is good for it and it responds accordingly.

I don't think enough emphasis is put on the importance of stretching our bodies and, as a result, up to ninety-five per cent of people who exercise don't stretch enough.

When we exercise we are working our muscles – pulling the fibres shorter in contraction and then lengthening them on release. This process can cause the muscles to become inflamed and tight afterwards, particularly if you are working hard. By taking some time to stretch the muscles out, you will aid muscle recovery and prevent injury. Stretching also helps prevent joint issues by opening and closing the joint space. You'll also see athletes stretching because it helps to improve performance and increase their range of motion.

The most important time to stretch is immediately post exercise. While stretching before working out can be beneficial, it can also lead to injury if you haven't warmed up first, so keep it gentle.

But I don't have the time!

Very few people literally 'don't have time' to exercise – it's just a matter of motivation and figuring out what's achievable for you.

First, you need to be honest with yourself and decide if you *really* don't have the time or if it's just an excuse. I'm guilty of this – when things are really busy with work it's easy to say that I don't have time for a run or that my time could be better spent elsewhere. What I have realised is that absolutely nothing will get done if I become unwell because I've neglected my body. I'm not going to feel good about myself if I've decided that I'm too busy to care for myself. If you resonate with this, it's time to make the decision to love yourself enough to dedicate some time to exercise – even a small amount is going to be better than nothing.

On the other hand, if you truly don't have the time to exercise, then you are going to need to rearrange some things to make the time.

But before you can make the time, you need to see where you are spending the rest of it.

Exercise – where am I spending my time?

1. Make a list of your daily schedule for every day over a week. Be specific – what time do you wake up, have breakfast and drive to work, what is your work schedule, how long do you spend commuting, what do you do in the evening, and more?

2. How long do you spend on each of these things? Be honest – it might surprise you.

3. Make a separate list of your priorities. From most to least important, list what is important to you. This may include family, work, exercise, meditation, reading, TV, education, hobbies and more.

4. Compare your priority list to your daily schedule – are you fitting in the things that are most important to you?

5. If you aren't, where could you save some time? Some ideas are:

   • Taking the train to work instead of driving and doing some work or reading on your commute

   • Going to the gym on your lunch break rather than sitting at a café

   • Getting up earlier in the morning to fit in some relaxation or exercise before work

   • Turning off the TV earlier in the evening and doing a meditation before bed (if you're worried about missing something, record it – you can always watch it in your allocated TV time later).

6. What can you eliminate from your schedule to make room for more fulfilling things?

7. How could you make things more efficient? Could you outsource or get help with anything that you have to do, like laundry, cleaning, or picking the kids up from school now and then?

Once you go through this exercise, you'll see that it really isn't too difficult to make the time to exercise a couple of times per week. If you're really time poor, then stepping up the intensity and doing shorter workouts is one way to benefit in a shorter amount of time. Consider doing three ten-minute stints a day. These are easily inserted into the day and are one way to increase your total daily exercise.

Finally, write a new daily schedule, including some exercise and other self-nurturing rituals like relaxation, cooking nutritious food or getting in the sun. If you want to get well and stay well, you'll need to put yourself first sometimes.

 TIP: *There is a great app called '7 Minute Workout Challenge' which takes you through twelve sets of basic exercises with rests in between and is a great one to get your heart rate up if you're time poor. There really are no excuses!*

Use your mind to succeed

Your mind is the number one determinant of whether you exercise or not. When you wake up for an early morning run, what are you telling yourself? Is it that you can't wait to see how good you'll feel afterwards, or that it's going to be so hard and you can't do it? Your self-talk is what will determine your success. So when you're getting started, promise yourself to only think about the benefits.

If you're trying to push your fitness to the next level then consider training with a friend to motivate you, or get a personal trainer who can encourage you to push your boundaries. Having that other person to push your limits is much easier than doing it on your own, where your thoughts can creep in and tell you that you can't do it.

Another way of avoiding this negative self-talk is to repeat positive mantras to yourself while you work out (for more info on mantras see Chapter 9). Try putting these phrases on repeat in your mind while you're jogging, cycling or trying to get stronger or go for longer:

- 'Fitter, stronger, healthier' – I use this one a lot when running
- 'I can do this' – Tell yourself you can, and eliminate the word 'can't' from your vocabulary
- 'Just do it' – Yes, this is a cliché Nike quote but it does ring true

When shouldn't I exercise?

Despite all of the benefits, there are some times when you should not exercise. These are:

When you are recovering from an injury (only do exercises recommended by your health practitioner), and

If you're about to get a cold or flu, or are feeling run down. In this case, avoid intensive exercise. Gentle exercise is still okay.

Make sure you ask your personal trainer, instructor or health practitioner about what type of exercise is safe for you if you are pregnant or have any health conditions.

Sitting is the new smoking

Even if you regularly go to the gym, being sedentary between your workouts can still lead to disease. In fact, researchers have found that those who live a sedentary life – that is lying or sitting for most of the day – are more likely to die from heart disease, Type 2 diabetes, and any other premature cause of death. So even though doing a thirty-minute jog is great, if you're remaining idle for the remaining 23.5 hours of the day, it might not be enough.

In an Australian study it was found that every hour of seated TV watching cuts twenty-two minutes from your life. Twenty-two minutes! By contrast, a study published in the esteemed British Medical Journal found that each cigarette a smoker had reduced their life span by eleven minutes. (You may not want to smoke while watching TV – the consequences would be horrific.) In other words, an hour of TV is worse for you than smoking a cigarette.

Now you might be thinking, *I don't watch TV. I'm not at risk*. However, considering that Australians spend an average of eighty per cent of their day sitting, you don't need to be a TV watcher to suffer the consequences of a sedentary lifestyle.

So what does it do to us? Sitting all day causes our systems to become clogged up. As many of our bodily processes rely on movement, inactivity leads to dysfunction of our organs and toxicity. This is a major cause of chronic disease, and researchers are starting to find that it is linked to other conditions too. Recently a study that came out of China examining hundreds of thousands of people and found that those with sedentary behaviours, such as watching TV or using computers, were twenty-five per cent more likely to become depressed.

So what's the solution? Besides swapping out your desk job for a place in the next Olympics, there are several things that you can do to modify your behaviour to get your body moving:

- Stand more often. Eat breakfast at your bench, walk around while reading the paper, and take a stroll while on the phone.
- Get a stand-up desk. Yes, you can stand up all day; you're just not used to it. Get a stool for breaks here and there.
- Sit on a fit ball instead of a chair. The movements make you activate your core and supporting muscles and you can bounce to move your body slightly.
- Take the stairs, not the lift. Or if you're on a really high floor, get out of the lift a couple of floors early.
- Park your car in the farthest spot from the shops, not the closest.

- Walk wherever you are able. If you can avoid the car by walking and taking public transport, this will mean less sitting time for you.
- Stay away from the TV. Or at least use the treadmill while you're watching it.

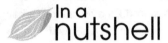

In a nutshell

Regular exercise is an essential part of getting well. Exercise moves blood around the body, ensuring nutrients get to where they're needed; it helps you metabolise fat and build muscle; it helps you detoxify; it increases your energy; and it even improves your sex life! If you don't think you have the time to exercise, it's time to look at your priorities and figure out how you can fit it in.

CHAPTER 11
ARE YOU NATURE DEPRIVED?

'Take two hours of pine forest and call me in the morning.'
–FLORENCE WILLIAMS

Are you spending the majority of your time indoors? In fact, if you think about it, you might not even have a window in your office, or access to natural light. Although this sounds like something out of a prison, this is the reality for many people who work in large offices, warehouses and city buildings.

We have evolved to be in and to interact with nature on a day-to-day basis, and multiple studies on the effects of being in nature on our health prove it. A Norwegian study published in 2009 found that the closer you live to nature, the healthier you're likely to be. In a 2011 paper, Japanese researcher Miyazaki concluded that stressful states could be relieved by forest therapy. It was found that people who gazed on forest scenery for 20 minutes a day had cortisol (stress hormone) readings 13% lower than those that only spent time in an urban setting. Meanwhile, researchers in Britain also found that spending just five minutes a day in nature had a positive effect on subjects' mental health.

It seems that connecting in with Mother Nature is no longer a hippie concept – hard science has shown that we need to spend less time in front of screens and more time outdoors.

Richard Louv, author of *Last Child in the Woods* and *Nature Principle*, hit the nail on the head when he said 'these days, unplugged places are getting hard to find'. We live in a world that is increasingly removed from nature, and as a result we have become 'nature deprived'. I believe that this lack of interaction with nature is a piece of the puzzle when it comes to the declining state of our health.

 TIP: *Some studies have found that surrounding yourself with images of nature or even just imagining yourself in nature can have a profound effect on your wellness. So bring nature to you by getting some indoor plants and putting them right near your desk or work station or wherever you spend the most time.*

So what are some of the other ways nature can benefit our health? The two main ones would be allowing us to produce vitamin D, and countering the effects of man-made electromagnetic fields.

Sunlight – yay or nay?

The sun is essential to your health – but how much is too much? There are mixed messages when it comes to sun exposure – we are told that we should avoid the sun to prevent skin cancer, but are also told that we need more sun to get our vitamin D levels up, with low vitamin D also associated with an increased risk of cancer.

The trick is finding the balance. I believe that we have now restricted our sun exposure too much and are suffering low vitamin D levels as a result.

There are over 20,000 research papers related to vitamin D – it seems that every week I am hearing about a new piece of research that shows yet another essential action of vitamin D. Just some of these benefits include:

- Preventing cancer,
- Preventing depression,
- Balancing hormones,
- Increasing sperm counts,
- Supporting thyroid health, and
- Regulating your immune system.

Under normal conditions we convert inactive vitamin D in the body to the more active vitamin D3 in the surface of the skin when it is exposed to sunlight. Most of this conversion happens in the softer surfaces of the skin – the inside of the forearms and your belly area. Now, unless we're at the beach it's unlikely that we get a good amount of sunlight on these areas of the body. No wonder we are deficient in this important vitamin! As well as this, research shows that the best time to get vitamin D from the sun is between 10am and 2pm – the times when we are taught to cover up to prevent cancer.

So what can you do? I recommend that you try and get at least fifteen minutes of unprotected sunlight every day, in the middle of the day. This could be two lots of 7.5 minutes where you put your forearms in direct sunlight. Or you could go and sit in a park on your lunch break.

As long as you do not cause skin damage then there is no evidence that you will increase your risk of skin cancer by doing this. Those with red hair and very fair skin may need to be cautious in summer though, perhaps by getting their exposure earlier in the day.

What else does sunlight do?

There is some really interesting research coming out about the other effects of sunlight besides vitamin D intake. It has been found that sunlight exposure can increase your nitric oxide production – a chemical that helps with circulation, keeping blood pressure low and preventing cardiovascular disease. There has also been some recent research in Europe showing that women who had less sun exposure throughout their lives had a higher early mortality rate than those who had more exposure. In the study, which examined over 29,000 people, it was found that the mortality rate in sun avoiders was two times higher than the group that received the most sun exposure. I believe that this is the first of a series of revelations to come about how our bodies use sunlight to stay in balance.

Electromagnetic radiation

The other area where connecting with nature has proven to improve our health is by countering the effects of electromagnetic fields (EMFs).

Although invisible to the human eye, EMFs are present everywhere. Naturally occurring EMFs, like that of the Earth or a thunderstorm, are harmless. Man-made EMFs omitted from things such as x-rays, mobile phone towers, and radio and TV broadcasters, however, can affect our health.

Because our bodies have an electrical charge, the EMFs we are exposed to everyday from Wi-Fi signals, mobile phone towers and electronic devices can influence the way that our bodies work, which could contribute to disease.

Work in this area is controversial; however, there are quite a few papers on EMFs showing effects such as changes on the cellular level and changes in health complaints. One example is a 2014 study published in the journal *Clinic Neurophysiology*, which investigated the effect of mobile phone signals on epileptics by testing their electrical brain activity on an electroencephalogram (EEG). They found that, when compared to the control group that wasn't exposed to any mobile signals, the group that was exposed to the signals experienced readable changes on the EEG. Although the changes were not large enough to cause an increase in seizures, the authors concluded that mobile phone communication systems do have the ability to slightly alter brain activity.

Studies on foetuses and foetal cells have discovered that those exposed to low frequency EMFs showed marked biological effects. One such study in the UK examined the effect of pregnant women living close to EMF sources and discovered that, by comparing 140,000 births, those who lived within fifty metres of high-voltage cables, overhead power lines, substations or towers during pregnancy were found to be more likely to give birth to babies of reduced average birth weights.

There are also reports that EMFs could contribute to conditions like cancer, cardiovascular disease, asthma, allergies and memory problems, but the research is divided – some studies show clear health effects and others show no change at all. Because of this division, the World Health Organisation states that the evidence on EMFs is inconclusive and therefore do not advise against their use. I would, however, err on the side of caution, as there are enough results out there to warrant further investigation.

My opinion is that there are certain individuals whose bodies cannot cope as well with the changes to their electronic fields that are caused by EMFs. As a result, it is wise to consider avoiding these fields, as it may help your body stay in homeostasis.

How to reduce EMF exposure
To reduce EMF exposure:
- Switch off Wi-Fi when not in use (including on your mobile)
- Avoid cordless phones
- Try not to have electronics in the bedroom
- Avoid carrying your phone on your body
- Switch your phone off when not in use

There are also several products that are available to offset electromagnetic radiation, such as certain crystals and devices that help prevent negative effects. Consider the bigger sources of

EMFs in your environment too – check you area for large overhead power lines, mobile phone towers and electricity substations.

Grounding for health

If EMFs can disrupt your body's electrical field, then how can you bring it back to balance?

An interesting area to look at is the effect of the Earth's magnetic field on our bodies. Studies have shown that 'grounding' or 'earthing' – when you have a connection with the Earth's surface – affects our bodies on several levels. On a basic level, it has been found that contact with the Earth causes a rapid decrease in electrical potential in our bodies. In simple terms, you could think of contact with the Earth as being able to defrag us. We know that when we defrag our computers they are less cluttered and work better, could this be the same for our bodies?

On a biochemical level, it has been found that earthing while exercising can:

- Reduce blood urea (meaning less muscle breakdown) levels,
- Reduce blood viscosity, which could help to prevent cardiovascular disease,
- Regulate cortisol levels, which are a major factor in how well we cope with stress, and
- Improve thyroid function.

More research needs to be done in this area, but it appears that grounding is just as important as sunshine, sleep and a good diet.

How to get grounded

When you put your feet or body on the Earth's surface – be it soil, rock or sand – it helps to stabilise your energy field. Simply sitting or standing on the Earth without rubber or plastic shoes on will help to keep you healthy. It's not that difficult to incorporate some grounding time into your day – sit on the grass during your lunch break, go barefoot when you hang out the washing, or eat your dinner on the grass outside during summer. A day on the beach might be just what you need to soak up some vitamin D and defrag your body.

If you can't get any 'Earth' action, look into a grounding sheet, particularly if you are stressed or have hormonal or thyroid problems. Grounding sheets have conductive thread which makes contact with your body and then goes out a window to be pegged to the ground, or plugged into the grounding hole of a power point, which ultimately ends up in the ground too.

Do they work? Well, an interesting 2004 study examined the use of grounding sheets on sleep, pain and stress. It was found that using the grounding sheets significantly improved sleep and self-rated levels of stress and pain. If you'd like to try one, search online retailers for 'grounding sheets'.

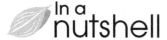 In a
nutshell

Our bodies have evolved to spend time in nature, and sunlight and being in contact with the Earth's surface has been scientifically proven to be beneficial for our health. Just twenty minutes a day in a natural environment like a park, backyard or courtyard with plants is enough to help your wellbeing. And exercising outdoors is a great way to kill two birds with one stone.

CHAPTER 12
THINK YOURSELF HEALTHY

'Your body hears everything your mind says.'
−NAOMI JUDD

We all know that eating the wrong foods, smoking and drinking too much can lead to disease. But what if you could think yourself sick? Better still, what if you could think yourself *better*?

The placebo effect is the most well known example of how our thoughts affect our health. The placebo effect was first mentioned in a paper in The Lancet, one of the world's oldest medical journals, in 1920. Scientists first discovered the placebo effect when they noticed that patients who were given a dummy treatment would get better, even though they had not had any 'active' treatment.

The placebo effect accounts for anywhere from eighteen to eighty per cent of patient recovery and traditionally placebo medicine was often prescribed to patients with good will, knowing that it was likely to have a beneficial effect. Even if we just use the lower figure, eighteen per cent is still a significant improvement considering all that had changed for the patients was that they thought they were going to get better.

This is why the practitioner-patient relationship is so important – part of the role of a practitioner is to inspire and paint a vision of a positive outcome for patients so that they will believe that they can get well. Unfortunately, with most GP visits being five to ten minutes long, there isn't much time to foster a meaningful relationship and I believe the patient suffers for this.

On the other side of the spectrum, there is also a documented 'nocebo' effect, which is where the patient has the negative side effects of a drug, even if they only took the sugar pill. The nocebo effect is also evident when patients' conditions worsen if they expect them to.

For example, in a 1999 study testing the effects of both placebo and nocebo effects, patients were administered a muscle relaxant or a placebo and were either told that it was a muscle relaxant, a muscle stimulant or told nothing about it. The participants that were told that it was a stimulant had significantly more muscle tension than the other participants, *despite* having received a muscle relaxant or placebo. Other studies have shown that people who are given decaffeinated coffee and told it was caffeinated experience physiological changes consistent with caffeine intake. Similarly, a 2006 study in the British Medical Journal found that proper adherence to placebos (meaning, patients taking placebos in the dosage and frequency prescribed for the real drug) was associated with decreased mortality.

By now you probably get my drift – whether you think something will make you better or whether you think you'll have negative side effects, what you expect to happen is likely to happen, regardless of whether you take the drug or the placebo.

I see the placebo and nocebo effects in my practice every day. Patients will most often get the best results in the beginning of treatment, when they are the most excited and motivated to make a change. I often have patients referring others to me even before their treatment has had time to work, simply because they feel so good! On the other hand, if a patient is worried about an adverse reaction to a herb, even if there is no basis for concern, I avoid giving them the herb as it is likely that they will experience the effect anyway.

The placebo and nocebo effects demonstrate that your mind is the most powerful organ in your body. It tells your body how to function, how to move, and what to feel. It can change the way that your cells function and it can change the way that your body experiences change.

And it can help you get well.

Dr Emoto's work[2]

The late Dr Masaru Emoto, author of *Messages from Water*, *The Hidden Messages in Water*, discovered that our thoughts can affect the structure of water.

In the mid-1990s, Dr Emoto began studying water by freezing it then looking at the crystals under a microscope. In the first study conducted, he found that when monks meditated over a polluted lake, the quality of the water crystals changed dramatically, going from a sludge-like consistency to beautiful crystal formations. Since then, multiple studies have been done along these lines and have found that the use of negative and positive words can actually change the crystalline structure of the water.

Considering our bodies are made of over sixty per cent water, these findings are astounding. Imagine if switching your negative thoughts to positive ones could change your health, and even the structure of your cells.

The impact of negative thoughts on your health

So we know from the nocebo effect that when you take a drug that you think will give you side effects, it is more likely that it will. It stands to reason that your own thoughts, feelings and expectations will affect your health outcome.

So could your negative beliefs be harming you? A study in The Lancet examined the death records of almost 30,000

---

2   www.masaru-emoto.net/english

Chinese-Americans and compared them to over 400,000 randomly selected white people. It was discovered that the Chinese-Americans would die significantly earlier than normal (by as much as five years) if they had a combination of disease and a Chinese birth year which astrologists consider ill-fated. On examination, the researchers found that the more strongly attached they were to traditional Chinese culture, the earlier they died. After excluding all other possibilities it was concluded that they died earlier because of their beliefs. In other words, they died younger because they believed that they were destined to have ill-fate.

Another interesting study showed that seventy-nine per cent of medical students develop symptoms suggestive of the illnesses they are studying. Dr Lissa Rankin, author of *Mind over Medicine: Scientific Proof That You Can Heal Yourself*, has described this term as 'medicalstudentitis'.

So what is it that you think about yourself every day? What are the thoughts, feelings and messages that you are giving yourself about your current health? What are your expectations of your future health? The answers to these questions may just become a self-fulfilling prophecy if you don't change your thoughts.

How to change your thoughts

The first thing that you need to do to change your thoughts is to observe them. Most of us, particularly when we are busy or rushing around, have no awareness of our self-talk. However, if you want to create lasting change, you need to pay attention to what is going on inside your head.

Your only job is to be an observer – listening without judgement. So if you are irritated or upset, you can observe this and acknowledge it without getting attached to the emotion.

Being able to observe yourself without attachment helps to reduce stress, anxiety and depression because you become less reactive to your thoughts and environment.

Exercise

Keep a small notepad and a pen on you for just one day. Observe your thoughts. Every time you have a negative thought, put a mark on your notepad, no matter how insignificant you think it is.

Negative thoughts include critical thoughts about yourself or others, thoughts that involve a negative outcome, worries and concerns. You'll be surprised at just how many negative thoughts arise throughout the day. Some examples of negative thoughts include:

- 'My ass looks huge in these pants.'
- 'I always feel tired in morning.'
- 'I'm not feeling well.'
- 'That guy is such an asshole.'
- 'F*@k it.'
- 'Oh shit.'
- 'I always get stuck at these lights.'
- 'I'm never going to get home on time.'
- 'I hate it when ...'
- 'I hate my ...'
- 'I can't believe they would ...'

Once you're aware of what's going on inside your head, you can make the choice to consciously change those thoughts. This isn't a process that happens overnight – you'll need to work to change your ingrained habits. However, there are some things you can do to help the process, such as focusing on the positive, changing your internal language, and practising gratitude more often.

Focusing on the positive

We know from the nocebo effect that if we think a drug will do us harm it is more likely to do so. So if you focus on the negative then you can attract a negative outcome.

However, by focusing on the positive you can attract more positivity into your life. This is the extension of the placebo effect – if you can get better just by thinking that you are taking a remedy, imagine what would happen if you started to think that good things were going to happen in all areas of your life.

In her book *The Intention Experiment*, Lynne McTaggart explores the connection between your intentions and outcomes. She discusses a number of experiments where scientists have proven that our thoughts and intentions can impact the way that our bodies work. In one study, it was found that when masters of Qigong applied positive intention to human fibroblast cells, the cell growth rates were increased by up to twenty-eight per cent after just two minutes. In another experiment conducted by American biologist Glen Rein, it was found that when doctor and healer Leonard Laskow focused his intention on cancer cells to normalise in petri dishes, the cancer cell growth rate reduced significantly. Now, this isn't a double blind, placebo-controlled trial, but this study does add weight to the body of evidence that is accumulating that our thoughts and intentions are more than figments inside our heads – they have the ability to change the way our bodies function.

These studies also support the law of attraction, which states that if you focus on something, you are much more likely to achieve it.

So, what do you want to attract into your life? Is it better health, more time with your kids, a better job? Think about what you want and visualise it every day – it's one of the most powerful ways to get it.

Some things that can help you to practice focusing on the positive include:

- Being around other positive people, or not buying into the negativity of others
- Igniting your sense of humour – try to see the funny side of challenging situations
- Practicing positive self-talk – focus on the good things
- Checking yourself periodically throughout each day to see if you've fallen back into old habits

Changing your internal language

The next step to changing the way you think is to start actively trying to change your self-talk. The list below gives some examples of how you might try to think of things differently:

If you're thinking	Try this instead
I can't do this	I like challenging myself
I'm really sick	I am getting better each day
I'm so tired	I'm working to improve my energy
I hate taking my supplements	These medicines are making me healthier
There's no way it will work	I am going to try and make it work
I don't have the time	I'll need to re-prioritise my time to make it happen
I hate feeling like this	This will change, it's only temporary
I always get sick	I'm getting stronger and stronger each day

You have free will, a choice to live and experience life any way that you want to. I invite you to step up and choose to be an active participant in the way that you think about yourself, your health, your happiness. Your choice will shape your future.

Gratitude work

Gratitude is one way of focusing on the positive. By focusing on the things we are thankful for rather than things that we don't want to happen, we can transition more easily through the darker times in our lives and feel happier and healthier.

Like many of the previous disciplines I've talked about, gratitude work has also been studied.

In 2003 researchers Edmonds and McCullough looked at the effects of keeping a daily or weekly gratitude journal on health and wellbeing. They found that people who kept a gratitude journal on a weekly basis exercised more, had fewer physical symptoms, were more optimistic about the upcoming week and felt better about their lives as a whole. Compared to other participants, people who kept gratitude journals were more likely to progress towards important personal goals, including those related to health. For those who kept a *daily* gratitude journal, the positive effects were even stronger, particularly in the areas of enthusiasm, determination, attentiveness and energy.

In another study, psychologist Dr Martin Seligman got participants to write a letter of gratitude to someone from their past; someone they felt they had never properly thanked for their kindness. The participants immediately exhibited a large increase in their happiness scores, an effect which lasted for more than a month.

I find this work amazing. By being grateful for the good things in your life you can truly change the way that you look at life, and experience profound benefits.

How to cultivate your gratitude

Gratitude can come in many forms, from simply thanking another person to letting them know that you are grateful for what they have done for you. It's not just about other people, either – it can be being grateful for having food on your plate or hot water, for getting to work on time or for a chance encounter. You can be grateful for having two legs to stand on, or for being able to exercise. We are often not grateful for something until we don't have it anymore – anyone who has broken an arm or leg knows just how much they appreciate it once they can't use it. Think of all the little things that make your life easier and be thankful for them every day.

To cultivate your gratitude, try these activities;

- **Keep a gratitude journal** – At the end of each day think of at least five things you are grateful for and write them down. You can also get various gratitude journal apps, which you can do easily on your phone.
- **Write a thank-you note or email** – Make it a regular habit to write to people and thank them for the positive impact that they have had in your life. This might be people from your past, or those who have made you smile on a day-to-day basis.
- **Get perspective** – Think about what your life would be like if you had to go without something, and then give thanks for the positive difference that it makes.
- **Practice mentally saying thank you** – As good things happen to you, mentally say thank you for them occurring. This is one really powerful way to hone in on the positive and is especially important in darker times when it is easier to focus on the negative.
- **Pray** – Some people find gratitude through prayer, which helps to bring to light the positive things in their lives.
- **Count your blessings** – Once a month, put a note in your diary to count your blessings. Make a list of twenty of the wonderful people/things/events in your life.

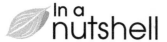 In a
nutshell

Your thoughts can change your health – so do you think that you're healthy, energetic and happy, or do you think that you're sluggish, tired and sick? You are what you think so it's time to start being aware of how you think and to start working to actively change it.

CHAPTER 13
SUPPORT OPTIONS

'The human body is the only machine for which there are no spare parts.'

– HERMANN M BIGGS

I'm thrilled you're reading this book and I hope it will help you get well and stay well, but sometimes just changing your diet and lifestyle is not enough. For most of you there will be times throughout your life when you will need some professional help to get your health back on track.

If you have any severe or unusual symptoms, the first place that you need to check in is with your doctor. A doctor is trained to diagnose and treat severe disease, so your GP is the one who can rule out anything sinister.

Now, if you visit your GP and they have told you...

a) There is nothing wrong with you,
b) That they don't know what is wrong with you,
c) That your symptoms are harmless and are nothing to worry about, or
d) That the treatment involved is severe and may cause harm...

Then it may be time to look for an alternate view, and this is where natural therapies come in.

The other case is when you have a condition that isn't as likely to be resolved based on diet and lifestyle alone. This doesn't mean it's impossible, just that I have observed that these patients also need some natural medicine to really get well. For these conditions, help should be found from a naturopath, acupuncturist or other health professional. This can be alongside your doctor's care or, for some patients, natural therapies may be the only intervention needed, depending on severity.

These conditions include:

- Amenorrhea (lack of periods)
- Asthma
- Autoimmune disease – Psoriasis, Ulcerative colitis, Crohn's disease, SLE, MCTD, rheumatoid arthritis, scleroderma, sarcoidosis
- Cancer (for any type you'll need the care of a doctor also)
- Chronic fatigue syndrome
- Chronic period pain
- Endometriosis
- Fibroids
- Fibromyalgia
- Hepatitis
- Lyme disease
- Parasitic infection
- Polycystic ovarian syndrome (if advanced)
- Recurrent migraines
- Severe acne
- Severe or chronic allergies

So what sort of therapists are out there?

Naturopathy and acupuncture

For most conditions that involve more than just body pain you can choose from naturopathy or acupuncture to get to the bottom of it. I will make no apologies for saying that I am a little bit biased and do like to send people to naturopaths first. As a naturopath myself, I know first-hand exactly how wonderful people can feel after getting this support, so a good naturopath is always a good first port of call. You'll get a really good understanding of what is happening with your health and what type of diet and lifestyle factors you will need to change.

In saying this, I do also work with a team of health professionals in my clinic and wholeheartedly recommend acupuncture as an alternative. Acupuncture is a whole body therapy that helps balance energies in the body and addresses the physical, mental and emotional aspects of health. Acupuncture comes from the Traditional Chinese Medicine framework, which involves the use of herbal medicines and dietary modification as well as acupuncture itself. Unfortunately, many acupuncturists in Australia only use part of this holistic method, which leaves gaps in their treatment. Naturopathy works extremely well alongside acupuncture in these cases, as naturopaths will cover the diet and lifestyle and prescribe herbal medicines which will assist with faster recovery.

Homeopathy

My experience with homeopathy is limited but for some this works wonders too. Homeopathy is an energetic form of medicine so it is great for those who are very sensitive. Homeopathy has recently come under fire from medical authorities who have touted it as 'quackery'. My opinion on this is that it seems pretty common sense that if thousands of people worldwide are using homeopathy with great results, then this should be the measure of success. Any medicine that helps people to live a more enriched life is worth using, and I have heard many positive accounts of homeopathy over the years.

Physical therapy

Now, if body pain is the main issue then you have several options. Chiropractors work by identifying and gently adjusting blockages in the spine. A good chiropractor will send you for x-rays and be able to give you a diagnosis of the problem and a treatment plan.

Osteopaths work more holistically, using more soft tissue and ligament work than chiropractors. In my opinion osteopathy and chiropractic can work equally as well if you have the right practitioner, although those seeing a chiropractor may benefit from massage in conjunction with their treatments.

Remedial massage can be helpful for those with body pain and is also great in combination with chiropractic and osteopathy. As well as releasing muscular tension and loosening up the body, a remedial massage can also help you to de-stress and unwind (depending on how knotty you are!).

Musculoskeletal therapy is like physiotherapy crossed with massage – these practitioners are awesome at diagnosing the cause of the issue and treating accordingly.

Physiotherapy is not something that I recommend often, simply because the feedback that my patients give me does not lend to its efficacy for long-term health. I believe this could be that many physiotherapists are caught in the 'medical model' with a focus on helping patients to recover from surgery or injury, rather than promoting wellness. There are, of course, exceptions to the rule and if you find a great physiotherapist then this might be the right avenue for you.

What about therapy?

So you've changed your diet, you're exercising, meditating and trying to think positively. But there's still something else that's not quite right. This is the part where I'm going to tell you that you might need therapy.

So before you think you need to go off and see a shrink, let me explain what I mean. All of us have emotional baggage that our subconscious minds carry around. For some of us, this baggage is causing problems for us now, even if we don't know it. In fact, most of the time we don't realise what might be affecting us now. This is because of our limited level of consciousness – we only consciously use five to ten per cent of our brains. The remaining ninety per cent is the subconscious, a place where we hide our deepest feelings, memories and experiences.

We are preconditioned to hold on to negative memories and feelings, simply because we're taught to repress our emotions when we're growing up. There are very few people who have been brought up to openly deal with emotions and instead they can lie buried in the subconscious, creating issues that we don't even know about. This means that dealing with this emotional stress is a skill that we often need to learn in adulthood.

There are many different ways to find out if there are any subconscious issues affecting your health. These modalities work on the underlying emotional and spiritual blockages that are causing you unhappiness and illness. Although it might seem a little 'out there' to some, I have seen this type of healing yield miraculous results for my clients. If you have a very stubborn condition that isn't responding to anything else, then an energetic healing session can really help to move things along.

Personally I have tried hypnotherapy, body talk, kinesiology, holographic kinetics, the life line technique, energetic healing and spiritual healing, to name a few! Each modality and individual therapist will have different techniques and insights to help you.

Hypnotherapy helps your body to get into a relaxed state where you can access the subconscious mind to identify if there are any issues. You can also use hypnotherapy to specifically look for a time in your life where a disease or bad habit might have originated.

A holistic counsellor or psychologist can also be of great help to many people, particularly when used with tools like cognitive behavioural therapy (CBT), emotional freedom technique (EFT) or mindfulness.

Kinesiology is also an excellent healing modality – but there are so many variations of kinesiology that they are hard to list them all. In particular, the therapists that work on emotional stuff as well as physical are really great.

Regardless of the therapy, most of them are centred on the acknowledgement of your emotions or beliefs and then a process to cleanse and release these beliefs so that they no longer cause issues for you. Spiritual or intuitive healing is also an avenue that you can take to see what is happening with your body on an emotional and spiritual level and is something I recommend regularly.

In my own journey of self-discovery I have learnt that really there is no end to the amount of healing that we can do. We are constantly growing, changing and experiencing new challenges and need support and healing so we can get the best out of life. Having a support team of qualified and experienced therapists can really help you to reach your full potential and can uncover issues that need attention.

Supplements

Like it says on the bottle, supplements should not replace a varied diet. Supplements are just that – a 'supplement' to your diet to increase nutrients in the body. You can never get your full range of nutrition from supplements as, in addition to vitamins and minerals, there are swathes of phytonutrients in foods that make up their complex nutritional profile.

Additionally, we don't fully understand the way that the nutrient profiles of natural, whole foods are balanced to include the right levels of nutrients in the right balance for optimum absorption and action in the body. As an example, while a supplement made from the components of green tea has some of the beneficial nutrients it contains, because we don't know how the various parts of green tea leaves work together to allow us to absorb those nutrients (in fact, there are nutrients in green tea and other foods that we don't even know about yet) a supplement made from individual compounds is unlikely to have the same benefits as the whole food. A supplement will therefore never replace an awesome diet. But they can be very useful for giving your body a boost.

So does that mean you should be taking a multivitamin, or other supplements, every day? Do you really need extra nutrients? It depends. It depends on whether you eat a totally organic dict, don't have any stress, have no environmental toxin exposure and take regular holidays to recharge your batteries. If this isn't you, then I bet that you'd benefit from taking a multivitamin, at least every now and then, to help give your nutrient levels a boost so your body can work the way that it is meant to. The trick here is taking the right type of supplement.

As you've probably already noticed, I'm a big believer of being under the care of a naturopath or nutritionist so that you are best guided to take what is appropriate for you at this stage of your life. Even if you just have one visit, a health professional can guide you towards some quality supplements, even if it's just a multi, which will give your body what it needs to function.

The problem with over-the-counter supplements

There are several issues that I have with people taking over-the-counter supplements. They are:

- They vary in quality depending on the manufacturer, price and raw materials;
- They could be in the wrong biochemical form, so you may not absorb them or utilise them as well; and
- Self-prescribing can lead to more imbalance in the body than you began with if you get it wrong.

Even if you know which nutrient to take and how much, each supplement is made up of different nutrient forms, which have varying degrees of bioavailability, absorption and action in the body.

I see it time and time again – patients come in, we assess their self-prescribed supplements and it turns out they need very little of what they have and what they do have is of poor quality or the wrong type. So, if you don't want to spend thousands of dollars throughout your life on supplements that aren't really making you healthier, it pays to make an investment in your health and check in with a professional.

Doctors and nutritional advice

I want to address an issue that I see sometimes – doctors giving erroneous nutritional advice. It is great that some doctors see the value of good nutrition (even if it is just about low iron or vitamin D), but the advice that is sometimes given can come from a place of no background knowledge about nutrition.

I see this a lot, particularly when prescribing iron and calcium. Unless your doctor has taken up post-grad studies in nutritional medicine, check in with a naturopath or nutritionist to find out which supplements are best to boost your levels.

Just the wrong damn product

Two of the most widely prescribed supplements are iron and calcium. These minerals must be in the correct forms to allow for good absorption through the intestinal wall. Unfortunately, the most widely-available and conventionally-recommended forms of these minerals are poorly absorbed and could even be harmful for your health.

Iron is often prescribed as ferrous sulfate or ferrous fumarate, which are both forms that are not well tolerated – causing constipation and digestive problems. This can cause problems with absorption and it can then sit in the gut and cause inflammation.

Calcium is important for the prevention of osteoporosis, and supplements are often recommended to ageing women to keep their bones strong. However, the leading supplement in Australia is made from calcium carbonate – the crappiest form of calcium that you could ever take. It's like eating chalk. Calcium carbonate has very poor absorption and is not a good form to keep calcium levels high. Use calcium in the form of calcium glycinate, calcium amino acid chelate, calcium citrate or calcium phosphate for better absorption.

TIP: *If your nutritional supplements are made by a pharmaceutical company, they probably aren't the best.*

Super food supplements

Super food supplements are a great addition to the diet to increase phytonutrient levels. They are often high in nutrients and have a good antioxidant profile too. However, they shouldn't replace a balanced and varied diet. See page 136 for more information about super foods.

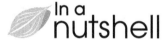

While changing your diet and lifestyle is a good start, it might not be enough to treat chronic conditions. Seeking help from health professionals can help give your body what it needs to heal.

CONCLUSION
IT'S NOW UP TO YOU

'Healthy is not an accident, a gift, or a rabbit's foot. It is a HABIT. It is a habit that will shape the bodies that we were born with, a habit that will support the genetic makeup we got from our parents.'
— CAMERON DÍAZ

I love this quote by Robert Brault – 'The way he treats his body, you'd think he was renting.'

You only have one body that will be with you into your old age. Your choices now will determine if your body will carry you into a healthy, self-sufficient future or if you'll end up in a nursing home. So are you going to treat your body like a rental, or are you going to be a proud home owner?

We've covered a lot of ground in this book and I hope that you've already made some plans to improve your health and your life. Here's a reminder of some of the most important foundations you'll need to get well and stay well:

1. Pay attention to your body and listen to what any signs or symptoms are telling you
2. Stay hydrated! Drink around two litres of water a day, every day
3. Chew your food well
4. Don't eat a food that makes you feel unwell in any way
5. Eat organic wherever possible
6. Avoid sugar and refined carbohydrates

7. Keep your coffee intake to one a day, in the morning
8. Drink small amounts of alcohol, but not too often
9. Avoid refined oils like canola oil, vegetable oil and margarine
10. Eat green leafy veggies every single day
11. Make fruit and vegetables the basis of your diet
12. Eat a varied diet of whole foods to get a wide range of vitamins, minerals and phytonutrients
13. Avoid canned food, soft drink and table salt
14. Make sure you're getting 8 hours a night sleep
15. Use only natural products on your body and in your home
16. Detox at least once per year
17. Get out in the sun for ten minutes a day to soak up some vitamin D
18. Spend time in nature to recharge your batteries
19. Train your brain to think positive thoughts
20. Practice gratitude in all areas of your life

If you're ready to own your body and treat it with the love and care it deserves, reading this book has given you the knowledge to do so. But knowing is very different from doing, and from here on it's up to you. Are you ready to take your health to the next level and make some significant changes in your life?

I implore you – love yourself enough to take the plunge and give your body what it needs to function at its peak. I promise you that making these changes will make you not only healthier, but happier as well.

Some days will be challenging, yes, and part of being well and staying well is persistence. But I don't expect that anyone to follow all of the guidelines in this book 100 per cent of the time – I certainly don't, and neither should you.

This isn't just another fad diet or short-term fix – this is your life, and creating a sustainable life is about balance. It's about nourishing your body with the wholesome foods it needs to keep you alive and well. It's about honouring your emotions and understanding the complexity of your mind and spirit and listening to your heart rather than your mind. It's about taking responsibility and loving yourself enough to do the right thing for your highest good.

And it's also about having fun. There is no need to be a raw, vegan monk who does yoga and meditates three hours a day! There is absolutely a way to find balance in this busy world, enjoying the things that you love without having issues with your health. Being healthy and enjoying things like wine, chocolate and coffee can actually go together. It's all about how often you have these things, and what you're doing in between to help your body stay healthy.

However, while moderation is key, there are times when you should really try to be a purist. If you are severely ill with conditions like cancer, autoimmune disease or anything that is causing major issues, it might be worthwhile being stricter with your diet until you're feeling well again. For some conditions, like severe candida, it is best to avoid alcohol and sugars completely. Likewise, people with anxiety or nervousness should avoid caffeine completely. And while detoxing, it is good to be a purist for a while so your body can recover.

It all comes down to awareness

Everyone is an individual. I have no set advice for every patient when it comes to their diet – this is why it's important for you to know your body, both how it feels when it's in balance, and how it feels when it's out of balance. Then you can use your own observations, combined with advice from your naturopath or nutritionist, to find the best balance for you.

Life will throw you ups and downs that will kick you in the butt and suddenly your good intentions will fly out the window. It comes down to self-awareness and persistence. The only way that you can prevent life getting the better of you is to observe yourself. What are the early-warning signs that your health is suffering? Are you beginning to notice some of those niggling symptoms coming back? Has your sugar intake shot through the roof?

Have you gone from green tea to grande lattes? Has your exercise routine come to a standstill?

These are all signs of dysfunction in one way or another; signs that you are not nurturing your body with what it needs to be well. Signs that either your mind, body or spirit is out of harmony and needs some lovin' to get back on track.

I'm hoping that by now you've already integrated some of the advice from this book in to your day-to-day life. If you haven't, it's time to get cracking and begin to make the changes that will ultimately decide if you are going to be happy and energised or exhausted and dissatisfied with life.

Now it's up to you. For some of you it may not be easy but, as someone on the other side, I can tell you that it's worth it.

RESOURCES

Diet resources

Micronutrients

Vitamins and minerals

Nutrient	Best sources	Main functions	Things that reduce levels
Vitamin A	Apricots Butter Carrots Cod Egg yolks Green leafy veggies Fish liver oils Halibut Kohlrabi Liver Mint Salmon Sweet potato	Essential for eye health Helps bone growth Immune function Keeps hair and skin healthy Needed for taste and smell Regulates metabolism	Alcohol Diabetes Diarrhoea Gall bladder issues Pancreatic problems Smoking Stress
B1 (Thiamin)	Asparagus Beef and lamb Legumes Nuts	Energy production Nervous system function Stomach acid production Regulates heart rate	Alcohol Coffee Diuretics Diarrhoea

Nutrient	Best sources	Main functions	Things that reduce levels
B1 (Thiamin) *(cont.)*	Organic liver Pork (free-range) Wheat germ Whole grains		Exercise High aluminium or copper Pregnancy Stress Surgery Tea
B2 (Riboflavin)	Avocado Beans Broccoli Currants Dairy products Eggs Organ meats Whole grains Yeast	Energy production Important antioxidant Metabolism Niacin (B3) production	Alcohol Diabetes Fever High cadmium or copper Oral contraceptive pill Smoking Stress Surgery Thyroid disease
B3 (Niacin)	Almonds Chicken Legumes Eggs Mackerel Meat Peanuts Salmon Sardines Sunflower seeds	Circulation Detoxification Mood balance Lowers blood lipid levels	Alcohol Coffee Diabetes Diarrhoea Fever High cholesterol High aluminium Smoking Ulcerative colitis

Nutrient	Best sources	Main functions	Things that reduce levels
B5 (Pantothenic acid)	Avocado Beans Brains Crayfish/ lobster Egg yolk Green veggies Liver Milk Mushrooms Oranges Royal jelly Sweet potato Whole grains	Adrenal health Energy production Metabolism Skin and hair health Wound healing	Alcohol Coffee High copper levels Pregnancy Stress
B6 (Pyridoxine)	Brewer's yeast Cereal Chicken Egg yolk Legumes Mackerel Oats Offal Peanuts Salmon Tuna Walnuts	Boosts progesterone Detoxification Energy production Fertility Mood balance Nerve health Red blood cell formation	Alcohol Coeliac disease Coffee Diabetes Pregnancy Tea
Folate (B9)	Beans Eggs Green leafy veggies Lentils Organ meats	Cancer prevention Detoxification DNA formation Fertility Mood balance Red blood cell production	Alcohol Antibiotics Coeliac disease Diarrhoea Gastric surgery High copper levels Pregnancy

Nutrient	Best sources	Main functions	Things that reduce levels
B12 (Cobalamin)	Brain Clams Egg yolk Herring Kidney Liver Milk Oysters Poultry Red meat Salmon Sardines	Cancer prevention Mood balance Methylation (detox) Nerve function Red blood cell production	Alcohol Bacterial overgrowth (dysbiosis) Coeliac disease Crohn's disease Diabetes Gastric surgery Helicobacter pylori infection High copper, lead or mercury Pregnancy Smoking Ulcerative colitis
Vitamin C	Black currants Broccoli Capsicum Citrus fruit Guava Kiwifruit Parsley Pineapple Potatoes Raw cabbage Rosehips Strawberries	Adrenal health Collagen production – keeps everything together Detoxification Immune function Skin health	Allergies Antibiotics Cancer High copper or aluminium Infection Oral contraceptive pill Pregnancy Smoking Stress Surgery
Vitamin D	Egg yolk Fish liver oils Milk Sprouted seeds	Bone strength Cardiovascular health Hormonal control	Alcohol Crohn's disease Lactation

Nutrient	Best sources	Main functions	Things that reduce levels
Vitamin D (cont.)	Sunlight on unprotected skin	Immune modulation Mood balance	Pregnancy Ulcerative colitis
Vitamin E	Almonds Beef Butter Corn Egg yolk Nuts Sunflower seeds Wheat germ	Antioxidant Cancer prevention Cardiovascular health Fertility	Alcohol Breast feeding Coeliac disease Diabetes Gall bladder issues Liver disease Low-fat diet Pregnancy
Boron	Almonds Apples Hazelnuts Raisins Tomatoes Peanuts Pears Prunes Soy beans	Bone health Growth and developments Regulates other minerals	Fluoride Magnesium deficiency
Calcium	Almonds Dairy Egg yolk Green leafy veggies Molasses Sardines Sesame seeds Soy beans	Bone density Cellular communication Fertility Hormonal signalling Nervous system function Stress management Teeth health	Excess phosphate intake (soft drinks, fertilisers) High protein intake High lead levels Lack of exercise Magnesium deficiency Pregnancy

Nutrient	Best sources	Main functions	Things that reduce levels
Chromium	Asparagus Capsicum Cheese Egg yolk Grape juice Liver Lobster Mushrooms Nuts Oysters Prawns Prunes Raisins	Blood sugar regulation Cognitive function Weight management	Diabetes Excessive refined grains and sugar High lead levels Strenuous exercise
Copper *Copper levels are often high due to it being in our environment. See Chapter 6 for more details.	Almonds Beans Crab Lamb Mushrooms Oysters Pecans Perch Pork (free-range) Prunes Sunflower seeds Whole grains	Connective tissue formation Energy production Gene regulation Red blood cell production Wound healing	Alcohol High sugar intake Pregnancy
Iodine	Fish Shellfish Squid Seaweed Turkey Eggs Himalayan salt	Thyroid hormone production Cognitive health Foetal development Breast health	Pregnancy Smoking Alcohol Oral contraceptive pill

Nutrient	Best sources	Main functions	Things that reduce levels
Iron	Apricots Beef Cashews Clams Liver Oysters	Detoxifies lead Mood balance Immune function Oxygen transfer Skin and nail formation Thyroid health	Blood noses Haemorrhoids High copper, mercury or lead Menstruation Molybdenum deficiency Pregnancy Recurrent bruising
Iron (cont.)	Parsley Pine nuts Pumpkin seeds Soy beans Sunflower seeds Wheat germ		Stomach ulcers
Magnesium	Almonds Brazil nuts Cashews Cacao Green leafy veggies Mineral water Molasses Parsnips Soy beans Whole grains	Energy production Mood balance Muscle relaxation Stress management Regulates blood sugar Relaxes nervous system	ACE inhibitors Beta blockers Coffee and tea Diuretics Excessive water intake HRT Oral contraceptive pill Pregnancy Stress Sweating

Nutrient	Best sources	Main functions	Things that reduce levels
Manganese	Almonds Beans Coconuts Corn Fruit juice Kelp Liver Olives Pecans Pineapple Sunflower seeds Walnuts	Blood sugar control Brain and nerve function	Diabetes High lead or copper levels Pregnancy
Molybdenum	Beans Butter Chickpeas Kidney Lamb Legumes Liver Oats Peas Pork Soy Sunflower seeds Wheat germ	Detoxification Mood regulation Nervous system health	High copper levels Fluoridated water Low zinc levels High protein diets

Nutrient	Best sources	Main functions	Things that reduce levels
Selenium *Selenium is depleted in Australian soil so food sources may not be high.	Alfalfa Brazil nuts Cashews Crab Eggs Fish Garlic Liver Mackerel Oysters Peanuts Tuna Whole grains	Antioxidant Breast health Cancer prevention Detoxification Metabolism Thyroid health	Alcohol Pregnancy Smoking Vitamin C deficiency
Zinc	Milk Beef Ginger Herring	Antiviral Detoxification DNA production Immune function Mood regulation	ACE inhibitors Anaesthetics B6 deficiency Breastfeeding Diarrhoea
Zinc (cont.)	Liver Oysters Sunflower seeds Pumpkin seeds Whole grains	Stomach acid production Thyroid health Hormonal balance Wound healing	Diuretics Excessive urination HRT Menstruation Oral contraceptive pill Pregnancy Stress Sweating

Other nutrients

Nutrient	Best sources	Main functions	Things that reduce levels
Bioflavonoids	Berries Buckwheat Citrus fruit Pineapple Kiwifruit Onions Pawpaw	Anti-inflammatory Cancer prevention Highly antioxidant Immune modulation	Diet high in cooked and processed food
Choline	Beef Chicken Collard greens Egg yolk Salmon Shellfish Tuna	Brain health Cell membrane fluidity Detoxification Liver health Mood balance	Pregnancy Prolonged tube feeding Vegan diets
Coenzyme Q10	Heart Kidney Liver Made in your body Nuts and seeds Sardines	Antioxidant Energy production Oxygenates the body	Statin drugs inhibit production of this important nutrient
Omega 3	Anchovies Cod liver oil Chia seeds Flaxseeds Mackerel Mussels Sardines Salmon Walnuts	Anti-inflammatory Brain health Cognitive function Cardiovascular health Eye health Hormonal balance Immune function Lipid control	Diet high in omega 6 and 9 fats Low bile flow/fat malabsorption

The oh-yeah list in more detail

While it's easy for me to say 'just eat your fruit and veggies', the variety of healthy foods available offer many amazing benefits. Read on to learn more.

Fruit - what they do for you

- **Apples** – An excellent source of fibre containing the bioflavonoid quercetin, which has potent anti-cancer and anti-inflammatory properties and immune-modulating properties.
- **Apricots** – A great source of iron with a good amount of fibre too.
- **Avocados** – An excellent source of healthy fats, protein and fibre. They also contain a good whack of B vitamins.
- **Berries** – These are an excellent source of vitamin C and a source of anthocyanins, which are anti-inflammatory, neuroprotective and help to regulate moods. Blueberries, blackberries, mulberries and cranberries are the best choices, with blueberries also containing resveratrol, which has anticancer and antioxidant properties.
- **Kiwifruits** – Kiwis are a powerhouse of antioxidants and contain enzymes that can aid digestion and decrease inflammation. They are one of the best sources of vitamin C and, if you eat the skin as well, they are an amazing source of fibre for great bowel health.
- **Figs** – Fresh or dried figs are an excellent source of calcium.
- **Lemons** – A great food for detoxification and alkalising the body. The skin contains essential oils which are immune boosting and good for your digestion.
- **Pineapples** – Pineapples contain heaps of vitamin C and bromelain – an enzyme that aids digestion, reduces inflammation, reduces allergies and has anticancer properties.

- **Pawpaw (papaya)** – Papayas contain the enzyme papain, which helps with digestion, reduces inflammation, reduces allergies and has anti-cancer properties. Papaya is one of the most easily digestible foods and is also a great source of fibre and vitamin C.
- **Pears** – One of the best foods for the treatment of constipation, they contain soluble fibre, which helps keep the bowel healthy.
- **Pomegranates** – The only food to contain punicalagin, a substance that helps your cardiovascular system. It has been found to reduce cholesterol, reduce blood pressure and prevent atherosclerosis (plaque).
- **Prunes** – Prunes are excellent for constipation due to their natural laxative properties, and are also potent antioxidants.
- **Red grapes** – A source of resveratrol – an anti-ageing compound that has been shown to activate antioxidant production in the body.
- **Tomatoes (red ones)** – Tomatoes contain a compound called lycopene, which has been shown to prevent heart disease and cancer.
- **Watermelons (red ones)** – Like tomatoes, watermelons contain a compound called lycopene, which has been shown to prevent heart disease and cancer. Watermelon also contains the amino acid citrulline, which has benefits in the cardiovascular system.

Veggies – what they do for you

- **Asparagus** – High in chromium, which can help balance your blood sugar and prevent diabetes.
- **Broccoli** – Broccoli has all of the cancer-preventing benefits of cruciferous vegetables mentioned on page 125, plus it's a great source of folate, calcium, vitamin C (when raw) and B vitamins. A truly magnificent super food!

- **Cabbage** – A fantastic source of cancer-fighting indoles and detoxifying sulphur compounds. The outer leaves are also high in vitamin A.
- **Capsicums** – One of the richest sources of vitamin C (when eaten raw) and is packed with antioxidants.
- **Carrots** – A rich source of beta-carotene which helps preserve eye sight. They have been traditionally eaten to improve night vision because of this.
- **Celery** – A fantastic kidney cleanser, especially if you eat the tops. It is alkalising and contains compounds that are anti-inflammatory and antioxidant.
- **Cucumbers** – Cucumbers contain silica, which helps to improve skin and hair health. They are very cooling and can help to cleanse your kidneys. Great for congested skin, eczema, dermatitis and anti-ageing.
- **Eggplants (aubergines)** – Eggplants contain the potent anti-cancer and antioxidant chlorogenic acid. As if that wasn't enough, eggplant peels also contain nasunin, which can inhibit tumour growth.
- **Mushrooms** – Mushrooms are super foods, particularly shitake and reishi, but even the humble button mushroom can boost immunity. They are high in B vitamins and other nutrients that are essential for health and a good source of protein.
- **Okra** – An Asian vegetable that has a high amount of soothing mucilage. Add it to soups and stews as a thickener that will improve digestive health.
- **Onions** – Onions contain a bioflavonoid called quercetin, which has anti-inflammatory and immune-modulating effects.
- **Parsnips** – These have more fibre than any breakfast cereal. They are brilliant for treating constipation and can help restore the good bacteria in the gut.
- **Peas** – A source of lutein, which helps preserve eye sight. They are also a great source of soluble fibre, protein and

phytoestrogens, which help to balance oestrogen levels in the body.

- **Pumpkins** – An excellent source of vitamin A, zinc and fibre. Eat the skin for a super antioxidant boost (great roasted).
- **Spinach** – A great source of chlorophyll, which helps to detoxify and cleanse the body. It is also a source of calcium, magnesium and folate. It's great for inflammatory conditions and is also a rich source of plant iron.
- **Zucchinis** – High in antioxidants, its intake has been associated with decreased risk of breast cancer and gastric cancer.

Properties of common herbs and spices

- **Basil** – High in essential oils that are antioxidant and gut-flora balancing. It is also a great source of iron.
- **Cinnamon** – A great source of chromium which can help to balance blood sugar and prevent diabetes.
- **Chilli (cayenne)** – A great circulation booster and can fight inflammation and pain.
- **Coriander leaf** – A great detoxifier. It can help your body to detoxify heavy metals and is a great source of minerals.
- **Garlic** – Garlic has so many medicinal actions that it's ridiculous. Garlic can improve circulation, prevent blood clots, reduce inflammation, prevent cardiovascular disease, reduce bacterial overgrowth in the gut and may even be antiviral and immune boosting. For the best effect on your gut, eat raw crushed garlic (crush and add to meals last).
- **Ginger** – A powerful anti-inflammatory and circulation booster. It helps to stimulate digestion and is a must for those who are cold in constitution, or experience poor circulation or cold hands and feet.

- **Mint leaves** – These are great for your digestive system, help to prevent wind and soothe the stomach.
- **Mustard** – High in antioxidants and helps to break up mucous in the body. It is great for anyone with sinus congestion or allergies.
- **Oregano leaf** – Contains essential oils that are antibacterial, antifungal and anti-parasitic in the gut.
- **Parsley leaf** – A powerful detoxifying herb. It is a great source of iron and helps to alkalise the body, reducing inflammation.
- **Pepper** – A great source of antioxidants and can help to improve circulation.
- **Thyme** – High in essential oils containing thymol, a powerful antibacterial and antifungal agent. Thyme is also great for any coughs or mucous congestion on the lungs.
- **Turmeric** – Turmeric is simply amazing. If I had to choose one super food this would be it. Turmeric reduces inflammation across nearly every inflammatory pathway in the body, helps to detoxify through your liver, improves circulation and helps with bile production from the liver, improving digestion. Eat it regularly, preferably with some oil to help with absorption of the active compound curcumin.

Nuts, and the amazing benefits you'll go nuts for!

- **Almonds** – Almonds are very alkalising, so they can help to keep inflammation down. They are also one of the best sources of calcium and magnesium, making almond milk a great dairy alternative.
- **Brazil nuts** – The richest source of the mineral selenium, which is needed to detoxify the body and support thyroid health. They are also a rich source of magnesium. Eat two to three per day for thyroid health.
- **Cashews** – A great source of iron and are a great alternative to cream in recipes. Make a cashew cream by simply blending cashews with water.

- **Chia seeds** – A great source of vegetarian omega 3, fibre and mucilage, which heals the gut. They are also a prebiotic, helping to feed the good bacteria in the gut. Soak them overnight for best results.
- **Flaxseeds (linseeds)** – A great source of vegetarian omega 3. They also have a soothing effect on the gut due to their mucilage content (like a soothing slime on the gut wall). Soak and blend them for best results.
- **Pepitas (pumpkin seeds)** – One of the best sources of zinc. They have been shown to help men's health, being beneficial for the prostate.
- **Sesame seeds** – One of the best sources of calcium. Tahini, or sesame seed paste, can be used in dressings, on toast with honey, in hummus and other dips and in smoothies for a great calcium boost.
- **Sunflower seeds** – These have more iron, kilo for kilo, than red meat. Sprinkle them in salads or in to stir fries at the end for extra nutrition and crunch.
- **Walnuts** – High in omega 3, they look like tiny brains and, funnily enough, are an excellent brain food!

Super foods

- **Acai** – Acai contains high levels of antioxidants and vitamin C to support immunity and prevent disease. Like blueberries, it contains anthocyanins that can help to reduce inflammation and improve cellular health.
- **Bee pollen** – Bee pollen is an amazing super food. It is rich in vitamins, minerals, amino acids and natural enzymes. It is immune boosting and antiviral and is said to be a restorative tonic.
- **Baobab fruit** –A newer super food, Baobab fruit powder is very high in vitamin C and antioxidants. It also contains soluble fibre, which is beneficial to gut bacteria.
- **Camu camu** – A berry from Peru that is very high in naturally occurring vitamin C and amino acids.

- **Chlorella** – Chlorella is an algae that has powerful detoxification action. It helps to detoxify heavy metals and contains high levels of blood-building and alkalising chlorophyll.
- **Cacao** –If you don't know what cacao is you'll be familiar with cocoa, the commercialised toasted form of the cacao bean that is used in chocolate. In raw, untoasted cacao you'll find higher levels of magnesium, B vitamins and theobromine – the antioxidant phytonutrient that has been shown to boost moods, improve circulation and increase energy.
- **Coconut** – Water, oil, everything! Coconuts are one of the most amazing foods on Earth. Any part of the coconut is beneficial for health, but here is what each part does for us:
  - **Coconut water** – A healthy, cleansing drink. It is found in young coconuts before the flesh develops. Coconut water is nature's sports drink – it is full of electrolytes that help hydrate your cells and provide fluid balance in the body. Interestingly, coconut water is so similar in makeup to human plasma that it was used as a transfusion during World War Two. Drink during and after sports and exercise, and while drinking alcohol and the next day to prevent a hangover.
  - **Coconut oil** – The oil is made from the flesh of the coconut and has an ideal blend of healthy fats. It is high in Lauric acid, which exerts antifungal, antibacterial and antiviral effects. The fats in coconut oil are metabolised quickly in the body and are much less likely to be stored as fat. This makes it an ideal fat for weight management. It is a very stable oil that can be used in cooking without risking damage to its structure.
  - **Coconut milk** – Coconut milk has some of the properties of coconut oil. It is also a good source of fibre, B vitamins and vitamin E. The canned variety does contain BPA, though, so don't consume too much of this.

- **Goji berries** – Goji berries, or Chinese gooseberries, have been used in Traditional Chinese Medicine for thousands of years for male fertility enhancement. More recently they have been found to be a potent source of phytonutrients that are beneficial for health. The phytonutrients in goji berries may have anti-cancer, anti-inflammatory and blood pressure lowering effects.
- **Green tea** – Green tea contains catechins, a powerful antioxidant that has been studied extensively. Green tea intake has been associated with cancer and diabetes prevention, improving the microbiome of the gut (more good bacteria), improving circulation and preventing cardiovascular disease. Most studies show that three cups a day are needed – drink in the morning and avoid if you are sensitive to caffeine.
- **Hemp seeds** – Hemp seeds have a fantastic essential fatty acid balance and are one of the best sources of plant-based omega 3. They are also an excellent protein source, containing all nine essential amino acids. This, combined with their high fibre content and good antioxidant profile, makes hemp the poster boy of super foods. But Australian consumers beware – at the time of writing this book hemp was sold only for 'beauty' purposes or animal food. This is quite ludicrous considering that the hemp that is used for food products has negligible amounts of THC (sorry, it won't make you high), and it is sold in a cracked seed form to prevent you from germinating it. If you're not in Australia, use hemp as you would chia – in smoothies, muesli or as a healthy addition to salads.
- **Maca** – Maca is a root from South America that is available as a powder form. It is excellent for your endocrine system – particularly your adrenals and ovaries or testes. Traditionally it is taken to improve stamina and enhance fertility. It has a caramel-like flavour – add to smoothies or sweets for extra nutrition.

- **Macqui** – Macqui is a super food from Patagonia, Chile. It has a very high antioxidant rating, one of the highest of any food.
- **Mesquite** – This Peruvian super food is rich in minerals and vitamins, particularly calcium and magnesium. You can use it in baking or throw it into smoothies.
- **Spirulina** – Spirulina is a microscopic spiral-shaped algae that is packed full of nutrients. It contains iron, calcium, zinc, B vitamins and chlorophyll. It helps with alkalising and detoxification. It also helps to clean and improve blood cell production.
- **Slippery elm** – Slippery elm is a herb that helps to soothe and heal the gut. It is recommended for anyone with digestive issues (especially reflux) and those who have a family history of bowel or stomach cancer. Take a teaspoon in water once per day, or add to smoothies. And remember to drink lots of water while taking slippery elm to prevent constipation.
- **Wheat grass** – Wheat grass juice contains vitamins A, E and K as well as vitamins B1, B2, B3, B5, B6 and folate. It is also high in chlorophyll, which helps to detoxify and build the blood. Great for anaemia, ulcerative colitis and other inflammatory conditions.

Examples of awesome diets

There is no perfect diet for everyone. However, here are some examples so you can see what a healthy diet might look like.

Example #1

Breakfast – Quinoa porridge with almond milk, berries and ground sunflower seeds.

Snack – Apple and ten almonds.

Lunch – Salad with baby spinach, tomato, sweet corn, cucumber, grated beetroot and sprouts with two boiled eggs.

Snack – Bliss ball.

Dinner – Pan-fried mackerel with steamed veggies and mashed sweet potato.

Example #2

Breakfast – Super food smoothie with rice milk, banana, maca, cacao, chia seeds, pepitas, and rice and pea protein powder blend (natural and sugar-free).

Snack – One boiled egg.

Lunch – Salad with roast pumpkin, baby spinach, goat's feta and pine nuts dressed with balsamic vinegar and olive oil.

Snack – Watermelon.

Dinner – Lentil Dahl with brown rice.

Example #3

Breakfast – Two poached eggs on wholegrain spelt toast with organic butter, avocado and wilted spinach.

Snack – Pineapple and five walnuts.

Lunch – Roast veggie salad with roasted beetroot, sweet potato and carrot tossed with rocket and capsicum with a lemon, olive oil and tahini dressing and fish (canned or fresh).

Snack – Bliss ball.

Dinner – Spaghetti bolognaise with organic mince, grated carrot, mushrooms, capsicum, onion, garlic herbs and pureed tomatoes (from glass jar) served with gluten-free pasta.

Example # 4

Breakfast – Homemade muesli with rolled oats, buckinis (sprouted dehydrated buckwheat), pepitas, sunflower seeds and flaxseeds with honey, berries, organic yoghurt and almond milk.

Snack – Brown rice crackers with hummus.

Lunch – Frittata with veggies served with green salad.

Snack – Large handful of grapes and four Brazil nuts.

Dinner – Organic roast chicken with steamed broccoli and roast beetroot, carrot, onion and pumpkin.

Detox resources

Easy detox plans

The following plans have been designed to give your body a respite from day-to-day toxins while delivering enhanced nutrition to help you heal and regenerate. To help detoxify, you'll need to pay particular attention to avoid the toxins described in Chapter 6, if you're not already doing this.

Novice – 10 days

This detox is for those who are just starting out and are not ready to commit to a longer program. I would recommend, however, that if you get through ten days and are feeling good to try and continue for a little longer.

Not allowed

- Dairy milk and cheese
- Wheat – including bread, crackers, cakes, biscuits and commercial cereals
- Added sugars (check the label)
- Coffee
- Black tea
- Soft drinks
- Fruit juice

Every day

- Start your day with a large glass of water with fresh juice of half a lemon or one teaspoon of apple cider vinegar.
- Drink two litres of water a day, minimum.
- Dry skin brush every day.

Day	Breakfast	Snack	Lunch	Snack	Dinner
1	Porridge made on water with almond milk, 1 tbsp LSA and organic berries.	1 apple and small handful raw almonds.	Green salad with rocket, baby spinach, cucumber, capsicum, tomato and 2 boiled organic eggs. Dressing olive oil and lemon juice.	Hummus with celery and carrot sticks.	Roast organic chicken with steamed broccoli, carrot, cauliflower and peas.
2	Organic sourdough spelt toast with avocado and lemon juice.	Date and cacao bliss ball.	Green salad with rocket, baby spinach, cucumber, capsicum, tomato and leftover chicken.	Guacamole with brown rice crackers.	Lentil and pumpkin Dahl with brown rice.
3	Smoothie with banana, berries, almond milk, chia seeds, maca and LSA.	Hummus and brown rice crackers.	Leftover Dahl with brown rice.	Bliss ball.	Cauliflower soup with lentils.
4	Omelette with onion, garlic, spinach, mushroom. Drizzled with olive oil.	Fresh juice with celery, carrot, beetroot and ginger.	Leftover cauliflower soup.	Pineapple and 4 brazil nuts.	Organic steak and steamed vegetables.

Day	Breakfast	Snack	Lunch	Snack	Dinner
5	Bircher muesli with berries and organic yoghurt.	Pineapple and 4 brazil nuts.	Green salad with rocket, baby spinach, cucumber, capsicum, tomato and 2 boiled organic eggs. Dressing olive oil and lemon juice.	Bliss ball.	Fish cooked in coconut milk with steamed green veggies and brown rice.
6	Spelt toast with avocado and lemon juice.	Guacamole and carrot/ celery sticks.	4 corn thins with salmon/ tuna, avocado, tomato and alfalfa sprouts.	Bliss ball.	Frittata with sweet potato, spinach and onion served with green salad.
7	Green smoothie with kiwifruit, banana, berries and kale plus chia seeds and LSA.	Fresh juice with celery, carrot, beetroot and ginger.	Leftover frittata with salad.	Orange and 4 brazil nuts.	Pumpkin and red lentil soup. Served with sourdough spelt bread.
8	Bircher muesli with berries and organic yoghurt.	1 pear and a handful of raw almonds.	Leftover pumpkin and lentil soup.	Hummus and brown rice crackers.	Organic roast lamb with steamed green veggies, roast beetroot and onions.

Day	Breakfast	Snack	Lunch	Snack	Dinner
9	Omelette with onion, garlic, spinach, mushroom. Drizzled with olive oil.	Bliss ball.	Green salad with rocket, baby spinach, cucumber, capsicum, tomato and leftover lamb. Dressing olive oil and lemon juice.	Organic yoghurt and berries.	Lentil and pumpkin Dahl with brown rice.
10	Spelt toast with avocado and lemon juice.	Hummus and brown rice crackers.	Lentil and pumpkin Dahl with brown rice.	Pawpaw with 4 brazil nuts.	Grilled fish and green salad with lemon and olive oil dressing.

Intermediate – 21 days

This detox plan will help to work deeper than the ten-day one and removes gluten as well as wheat to help with further gut healing.

Not allowed

- Dairy milk and cheese
- Wheat – including bread, crackers, cakes, biscuits, commercial cereals
- Gluten – no rye, spelt, khorasan (kamut) or barley
- Added sugars (check the label)
- Coffee
- Black tea
- Soft drinks
- Fruit juice
- No red meat or chicken for the first ten days

Every Day
- Start your day with a large glass of water with fresh juice of half a lemon or one teaspoon apple cider vinegar.
- Drink two litres of water a day, minimum.
- Dry skin brush every day.

Example Diet
You can mix and match and add anything else in as long as it fits with the guidelines.

Day	Breakfast	Snack	Lunch	Snack	Dinner
1	Quinoa porridge made on water with almond milk, 1 tbsp LSA and organic berries and coconut oil.	1 apple and small handful raw almonds.	Green salad with rocket, baby spinach, cucumber, capsicum, tomato and 2 boiled organic eggs. Dressing olive oil and lemon juice.	Hummus with celery and carrot sticks.	Corn fritters with salad of baby spinach, tomato, capsicum, cucumber, sprouts. Lemon juice and olive oil dressing.
2	Gluten-free bircher muesli with berries and organic yoghurt.	Date and cacao bliss ball.	Leftover corn fritter and salad.	Guacamole with brown rice crackers.	Lentil and pumpkin Dahl with brown rice.

Day	Breakfast	Snack	Lunch	Snack	Dinner
3	Smoothie with banana, berries, almond milk, chia seeds, maca and LSA.	Hummus and brown rice crackers.	Leftover Dahl with brown rice.	Bliss ball.	Cauliflower soup with lentils.
4	Omelette with onion, garlic, spinach, mushroom. Drizzled with olive oil.	Fresh juice with celery, carrot, beetroot and ginger.	Leftover cauliflower soup.	Pineapple and 4 brazil nuts.	Quinoa tabouli salad with 2 poached eggs.
5	Gluten-free bircher muesli with berries and organic yoghurt.	Pineapple and 4 brazil nuts.	Green salad with rocket, baby spinach, cucumber, capsicum, tomato and 2 boiled organic eggs. Dressing olive oil and lemon juice.	Bliss ball.	Fish cooked in coconut milk with steamed green veggies and brown rice.

Day	Breakfast	Snack	Lunch	Snack	Dinner
6	Quinoa porridge made on water with almond milk, 1 tbsp LSA and organic berries and coconut oil.	Guacamole and carrot/celery sticks.	4 corn thins with salmon/tuna, avocado, tomato and alfalfa sprouts.	Bliss ball.	Frittata with sweet potato, spinach and onion served with green salad.
7	Green smoothie with kiwifruit, banana, berries and kale plus chia seeds and LSA.	Fresh juice with celery, carrot, beetroot and ginger.	Leftover frittata with salad.	Orange and 4 brazil nuts.	Pumpkin and red lentil soup. Served with sourdough spelt bread.
8	Gluten-free toasted muesli with berries and organic yoghurt.	1 pear and a handful of raw almonds.	Leftover pumpkin and lentil soup.	Hummus and brown rice crackers.	Corn fritters with green salad.

Day	Breakfast	Snack	Lunch	Snack	Dinner
9	Omelette with onion, garlic, spinach, mushroom. Drizzled with olive oil.	Bliss ball.	Green salad with rocket, baby spinach, cucumber, capsicum, tomato and some cooked chickpeas or beans. Dressing olive oil and lemon juice.	Organic yoghurt and berries.	Lentil and pumpkin Dahl with brown rice.
10	Live tropical porridge.	Hummus and brown rice crackers.	Lentil and pumpkin Dahl with brown rice.	Pawpaw with 4 brazil nuts.	Grilled fish and green salad with lemon and olive oil dressing.
11	Green smoothie with kiwifruit, banana, berries and kale plus chia seeds and LSA.	1 boiled egg and chopped carrot, celery and capsicum sticks.	Vegetable salad with cup legumes.	Bliss ball.	Quinoa tabouli salad with 2 poached eggs.

Day	Breakfast	Snack	Lunch	Snack	Dinner
12	Corn fritters with smashed avocado.	Pawpaw with 4 brazil nuts.	Quinoa tabouli salad with 1 boiled egg or cup legumes.	Hummus and brown rice crackers.	Cauliflower soup with lentils.
13	Smoothie with banana, berries, almond milk, chia seeds, maca and LSA.	1 boiled egg and chopped carrot, celery and capsicum sticks.	Cauliflower soup with lentils.	Guacamole with brown rice crackers.	Quinoa and Mexican beans.
14	Quinoa porridge made on water with almond milk, 1 tbsp LSA and organic berries and coconut oil.	Fresh juice with celery, carrot, beetroot and ginger.	4 corn thins with salmon/ tuna, avocado, tomato and alfalfa sprouts.	Pawpaw with 4 brazil nuts.	Organic steak and steamed vegetables.

Day	Breakfast	Snack	Lunch	Snack	Dinner
15	Fresh juice with celery, carrot, beetroot and ginger. Plus 1 boiled egg.	Pawpaw or pineapple with 4 Brazil nuts.	Green salad with rocket, baby spinach, cucumber, capsicum, tomato and some cooked chickpeas or beans. Dressing olive oil and lemon juice.	Hummus and brown rice crackers.	Frittata with sweet potato, spinach and onion served with green salad.
16	Green smoothie with kiwifruit, banana, berries and kale plus chia seeds and LSA.	Guacamole with brown rice crackers.	Frittata with sweet potato, spinach and onion served with green salad.	Bliss ball.	Roast organic chicken with steamed broccoli, carrot, cauliflower and peas.
17	Quinoa porridge made on water with almond milk, 1 tbsp LSA and organic berries and coconut oil.	Hummus and brown rice crackers.	Green salad with rocket, baby spinach, cucumber, capsicum, tomato and leftover chicken.	1 boiled egg and chopped carrot, celery and capsicum sticks.	Quinoa tabouli salad with 2 poached eggs.

Day	Breakfast	Snack	Lunch	Snack	Dinner
18	Live tropical porridge.	Guacamole with brown rice crackers.	Quinoa tabouli salad with 1 boiled egg or cup legumes.	Green smoothie with kiwifruit, banana, berries and kale plus chia seeds and LSA.	Lentil Dahl with brown rice.
19	Fresh juice with celery, carrot, beetroot and ginger. Plus 1 boiled egg.	Watermelon and 4 brazil nuts.	Green salad with rocket, baby spinach, cucumber, capsicum, tomato and some cooked chickpeas or beans. Dressing olive oil and lemon juice.	Hummus and brown rice crackers.	Organic steak and steamed vegetables.
20	Green smoothie with kiwifruit, banana, berries and kale plus chia seeds and LSA.	Bliss ball.	4 corn thins with boiled eggs, avocado, baby spinach and cucumber.	Fresh juice with celery, carrot, beetroot and ginger.	Organic roast lamb with steamed green veggies, roast beetroot and onions.

Day	Breakfast	Snack	Lunch	Snack	Dinner
21	Quinoa porridge made on water with almond milk, 1 tbsp LSA and organic berries and coconut oil.	Guacamole with brown rice crackers.	Vegetable salad with cup legumes.	Hummus and brown rice crackers.	Green salad with rocket, baby spinach, cucumber, capsicum, tomato and some cooked chickpeas or beans. Dressing olive oil and lemon juice.

Advanced – 30+ days

This detox builds on the twenty-one-day detox by including more juices and smoothies and eliminating meat for a little longer. You can use the meal plan from the twenty-one day detox – by the time you get to day 21 you'll have a really good handle on how to continue from there.

Not Allowed

- Dairy milk and cheese
- Wheat – including bread, crackers, cakes, biscuits, commercial cereals
- Gluten – no rye, spelt, khorasan (kamut) or barley
- Added sugars (check the label)
- Coffee
- Black tea
- Soft drinks
- Fruit juice
- No red meat or chicken for the first fourteen days

Every Day

- Start your day with a large glass of water with fresh juice of half a lemon or one teaspoon apple cider vinegar.
- Drink two litres of water a day, minimum.
- Dry skin brush every day.
- Two tablespoons of chia gel.
- Try having at least one super food smoothie or fresh vegetable juice per day to pump up your nutrition.
- Try to avoid meat for the first two weeks of the detox.

Detox recipes

Breakfast recipes

Quinoa porridge

Quinoa is an ancient grain originating in South America. It is gluten-free, high in protein and calcium and is a complex carbohydrate. I recommend making this porridge on Sunday and reheating it in the morning for a quick and delicious breakfast!

Ingredients
1 cup quinoa
2 cups water
1 cup rice milk or full-fat organic dairy milk
1 apple or pear – diced
1 tsp cinnamon
Pinch Celtic sea salt
1 cup chopped walnuts
Honey or pure maple syrup to serve

Method
1. Soak quinoa for at least three hours in water (or overnight). Discard water and rinse well using a fine sieve.
2. In a pot add rinsed quinoa, water and cinnamon. Bring to the boil then reduce heat and simmer for 15 minutes.
3. Add milk and apple to pot and continue to simmer for another 15 minutes, stirring occasionally.
4. Remove from stove and rest for 10 minutes. This will allow the porridge to thicken.

5. Serve while hot or put in a container in the fridge for later use. To reheat, put porridge in a saucepan with a little water or milk.

6. Serve hot with ¼ cup chopped walnuts and around a tsp of honey or maple syrup.

7. Enjoy!

The best gluten-free toasted muesli recipe

The problem with most muesli is that it is loaded with sugar and preservatives. Another issue is that toasting muesli with nuts and seeds makes the good oils in the nuts turn into trans fats, reducing their benefits. Do not despair – there is an alternative – my homemade gluten-free muesli!

This muesli is high in protein, gluten-free and contains alkaline grains and seeds, making it less acid forming than most muesli. Enjoy!

Ingredients

2 cups puffed amaranth

2 cups puffed millet

2 cups puffed buckwheat

½ cup raw honey (warmed if thick)

¼ cup macadamia oil (or coconut oil)

2 tsp cinnamon

1 tsp natural vanilla essence (optional)

½ cup pepitas

½ cup sunflower seeds

½ cup chopped almonds

¼ cup chia seeds

Methods

1. Preheat your oven to 160 degrees Celsius.
2. In a large baking tray/dish, add the amaranth, millet and buckwheat.
3. In a small bowl mix together the honey (warmed if thick), macadamia or coconut oil, cinnamon and vanilla essence.
4. Add honey mix to dry mix and combine well using the back of a large spoon. The mixture should be have a light and even coat all over with no clumps of honey.
5. Place tray in oven and bake for 10 minutes. Turn mix over a few times with a spoon and bake for a further 10 minutes.
6. Remove from oven and allow to cool.
7. Once cool add the nuts and seeds. Combine well and place in an airtight glass jar for storage. Serve with fresh berries or figs and yoghurt.

Bircher muesli

Bircher muesli is a great way to have your muesli. It involves soaking the muesli in yoghurt or apple juice overnight to soften it.

In a glass or stainless steel container put natural, sugar-free muesli and enough of any of the following (or a combination of) to fully cover it.

- Organic probiotic yoghurt
- Cold-pressed apple juice
- Rice or almond milk

You can also add grated apple, frozen berries and any super food you like. This usually lasts about a week in the fridge, so is great if you're time poor. Eat it for breakfast but also consider it for a healthy snack.

Raw live tropical porridge

Ingredients
Nut mix (will last for 4 servings):
2tbsp raw almonds
2tbsp pepitas
2tbsp sunflower seeds
2tbsp flax seeds or chia seeds
Fruit for one person:
½ ripe mango, finely chopped
¼ medium pawpaw, finely chopped
1 inch slice pineapple, peeled and finely chopped
1 tbsp desiccated coconut

Method

1. Soak all nuts and seeds in water overnight. Drain with a fine sieve and rinse well.
2. In a blender, place half of the soaked nuts and seeds and 1 cup of water. Blend on high until smooth.
3. Place the rest of the soaked nuts and seeds in the blender. Blend on low until nuts are finely chopped but still visible in milk. Mixture should be a runny thick consistency, but it is not essential.
4. Add 3 tbsp of nut mix and coconut to fruit and stir through. Enjoy immediately.
5. Place leftover nut mix in an airtight container in the fridge for up to four days.

Cacao, maca and banana super food smoothie

This smoothie makes a great breakfast or snack, and takes minutes to prepare. It works best if you peel and freeze the banana, to give it a thicker consistency.

Ingredients

¼ cup pre-soaked nuts (cashews, walnuts, almonds, etc.)

1 tbsp Lecithin granules (optional, make sure it is non-GMO)

1 rounded tsp maca

1 tbsp ground raw cacao powder

Cold water as needed – probably 1 cup

2 large peeled and frozen bananas, sliced (or fresh banana and ice)

Method

1. Place all ingredients in blender.
2. Blend until smooth and creamy. Add extra water if too thick and blend again.
3. Scrape into a tall glass and drink immediately.

Hearty scrambled eggs

This breakfast will give you sustained energy release, being high in protein and nutrients. Change ingredients to your liking but try to always include onion or garlic as they are great for the liver. Serve with dark rye or organic sourdough bread topped with avocado or tahini, or have on its own.

Serves 2

Ingredients

4 Organic Eggs

1/4 cup rice, oat, or organic dairy milk

Small handful fresh herbs (basil, thyme, oregano, rosemary all work well) or 1 tsp dried herbs

1 large garlic clove minced

Sea or Himalayan salt and pepper

1 onion diced

1/2 zucchini diced

1/4 capsicum diced

4 average mushrooms roughly chopped

1/2 cob fresh corn removed off cob

1 tbsp coconut, olive or rice bran oil

Method

1. In a bowl, whisk eggs with a fork until well mixed. Add milk, herbs, garlic, salt and pepper and whisk to combine.

2. In a small heavy based frying pan heat oil on medium heat. Add chopped vegetables and fry until lightly cooked through.

3. Add egg mix and stir through. Using an egg flip, lift and turn occasionally from bottom of pan until cooked through. Do not turn too frequently unless you want your eggs crumbly.

4. Eat on its own or serve with rye, kamut, spelt or sourdough bread topped with avocado.

Lunch and dinner recipes

Cauliflower soup

this is a great recipe to whip up at the last minute and is wheat, dairy and sugar-free. It's perfect for detoxifying due to the high levels of indoles and sulphur compounds in the ingredients, which help to cleanse your body.

Ingredients

1 whole cauliflower, roughly chopped

1 small sweet potato, roughly chopped

2 small potatoes (skin on), roughly chopped

4 celery tops (the leafy bits), chopped finely

2 onions diced

½ cup split red lentils

1 tbsp rice bran oil

1 ½ tsp Celtic sea salt or Himalayan salt

1 tbsp mixed dried herbs

Method

1. In a large pot, fry onion with herbs and celery tops until softened.

2. Add remaining ingredients, and then add enough filtered water to cover.

3. Bring to the boil, then reduce heat and simmer for 15–20 minutes.

4. Let cool slightly and blend with a stick blender (be careful not to splash yourself).

Quinoa tabouli

This a great spin on traditional tabouleh which normally uses bulgur wheat. This version can be enjoyed by those with gluten sensitivity and is this recipe is great for alkalising and detoxification.

Ingredients

1 cup quinoa – pre-soaked and rinsed well

2 cups water

½ cup freshly squeezed lemon juice

1/3 cup cold-pressed olive oil

3 tomatoes, finely diced

1 large bunch parsley, finely chopped

2 tbsp fresh mint, finely chopped

1 bunch shallots, finely chopped

A pinch good-quality salt

Method

1. Place quinoa in a saucepan with water. Bring to the boil then reduce heat, cover and simmer for 10 – 15 minutes or until water has absorbed and edges separate off quinoa grains.

2. Place all other ingredients in a large bowl. Once quinoa is cooled, add to mix and stir through until well combined.

3. Tabouleh tastes better if you let it sit overnight to let the flavours infuse. Remove from fridge prior to serving and serve at room temperature.

Vegetable salad

If you hate leafy cold salads then this is for you! This simple salad tastes great and can be had on its own or as a side to a meal.

Ingredients

4 handfuls of vegetables – broccoli, carrot, cabbage, cauliflower, parsnip, Brussels sprouts, peas – anything you like!

Balsamic vinegar

Cold-pressed olive or macadamia oil

¼ cup sunflower seeds or pepitas

Himalayan salt and pepper to taste

Method

1. Chop all vegetables up into small pieces and put in a steamer pot on the stove.

2. Steam until just done, and still a little firm.

3. Put veggies in a large bowl. Add seeds, a good splash of balsamic and a large glug of olive oil.

4. Season with salt and pepper.

5. Serve hot or cold.

6. For different flavours, add some minced garlic or chopped herbs in with the balsamic and oil. Serve with a can of salmon or some legumes for a quick lunch!

Corn fritters

These fritters are a great option for breakfast or for lunch and dinner served with salad.

Ingredients

2 cobs fresh corn – kernels removed off the cob

½ onion, finely diced

½ red capsicum, finely diced (you can substitute any other vegetable here)

1 clove garlic, crushed

2 eggs, beaten

1 tbsp buckwheat or rice flour

Salt and pepper to taste

Coconut oil or butter, for frying

Method

1. Put ingredients in a large bowl and mix together well.

2. Heat up a frying pan and add a little coconut oil or butter.

3. Spoon the mixture into the pan, around 2 tbsp per fritter.

4. Cook for 1 – 2 minutes and then turn using a spatula.

5. Serve with some Himalayan salt and smashed avocado.

Warm sweet potato and asparagus salad

warm salads are a great tasting alternative to your traditional cold raw salads, and there are many ways to have them. Try using cooked potato, parsnip, pumpkin, beans and broccoli.

Ingredients

1 small sweet potato, diced into small cubes

3 asparagus spears, chopped in pieces

¼ red onion, diced finely

½ handful baby spinach

1 small clove garlic, crushed

Fresh basil leaves, chopped

1 tbsp pepitas or sunflower seeds

Sea salt and pepper to taste

Dressing

1 tbsp probiotic yoghurt (Jalna)

½ tbsp stone ground tahini

Squeeze of lemon juice

¼ tsp cinnamon

Method

1. Steam sweet potato until soft, then add asparagus and cook for another minute.

2. Place the onion, spinach, garlic, basil, salt and pepper in a bowl. Add the hot vegetables and stir gently. Add the premixed dressing and pepitas and stir through gently.

3. Serve immediately.

Lentil and mushroom soup

i love lentils. Although they take a long time to cook this soup is very easy. It is a great source of iron and protein – enjoy!

Ingredients

1 cup green or brown lentils

2 large onions, finely diced

1 small bunch fresh thyme, or 1 tbsp dried thyme

2 large Portobello mushrooms (about the size of your hand), diced

4 tomatoes, diced

1 red capsicum, diced

1tbsp butter or rice bran oil

Filtered water

Sea salt and pepper

Directions

1. Cover lentils with water and soak for 24 hours. Discard water, rinse and place in a pot with 4 cups of water. Bring to the boil then simmer for 90 minutes with the lid on.

2. In a large saucepan, fry onions and thyme in butter or oil until softened. Add mushrooms, tomato and capsicum. Cook on low for 10 minutes, stirring frequently.

3. Add lentils (and the water they were cooked in), plus 1 extra cup of water. Bring to the boil then reduce heat and simmer for 15-20 minutes. Add sea salt and pepper to taste.

4. Take off heat and allow to cool for 10 minutes. With a stainless steel stick blender, blend to desired consistency.

5. Serve with spelt sourdough bread drizzled with olive oil.

Lamb koftas with chickpea mash

this meal is very high in protein and a great source of iron. Adding some other steamed vegetables such as broccoli, Brussels sprouts and beans can help to make this a complete meal.

Ingredients

250g lean lamb mince (preferably organic)

1 onion, finely chopped

I tbsp chopped fresh coriander

1 tbsp chopped fresh parsley

½ tsp ground coriander seeds

¼ tsp chilli powder

Sea salt and pepper to taste

Chickpea mash

1tbsp extra virgin olive oil

2 garlic cloves, chopped

1 cup cooked chickpeas

50ml rice, oat or Bonsoy milk

Pepper

2tbsp chopped coriander

Directions

1. Put the lamb, onions, herbs, spices, salt and pepper in a food processor. Process until thoroughly combined. If you do not have a food processor, chop ingredients as finely as you can and mix thoroughly.

2. Divide the mixture into 8 portions, and using wet hands shape each portion into a sausage shape around a wooden skewer (you must soak wooden skewers in water for at least 2 hours prior to use to prevent burning). Cover and chill in the refrigerator for 30 minutes.

3. Preheat a griddling pan or barbecue (or heavy based saucepan) and brush with a little oil. Cook the skewers, turning occasionally, for 10 minutes or until browned on all sides and cooked through.

4.   For the chickpea mash, heat the oil in saucepan and gently fry garlic for 2 minutes. Add the chickpeas and milk and heat through for a few minutes. Transfer into a food processor or blender and process until smooth. Season to taste with sea salt and pepper and stir through fresh coriander.

5.   Serve the koftas with mash and steamed green veggies on the side

Other recipes

Prune and orange muffins

This is my go-to healthy muffin recipe. The sweetness comes from the prunes and orange juice and they are loaded with fibre from the prunes, spelt flour and oat bran. If you're not passing a bowel movement every day, these would be a great inclusion in your diet.

Ingredients

280g pitted prunes, roughly chopped (preservative-free)

1 cup freshly squeezed orange juice

Grated rind of 1 orange

¼ cup water

¼ vanilla pod, scraped or 1 tsp natural vanilla essence

40g organic butter and 40g coconut oil (or you can use rice bran or macadamia oil)

½ tsp bicarbonate soda (aluminium free)

¼ cup rice milk or almond milk

1 tbsp honey

2 large or 3 small eggs, lightly beaten

2 cups wholegrain spelt flour

1/4 cup oat bran

3tsp baking soda

Method

1. Preheat oven to 190 degrees Celsius and grease a 12-hole muffin tin with oil and flour.

2. In a small saucepan, place the prunes, orange juice and rind, vanilla, water and butter/oils. Bring to the boil then reduce heat and simmer for 3–4 minutes.

3. Turn off heat and allow to cool slightly, then add bicarbonate soda and stir through.

4. In a bowl, sift flour and baking soda. Add oat bran and make a well in the middle.

5. To the prune mix, add honey and rice milk. Stir through. Once the mix is cool enough to touch, stir through egg yolks.

6. Add wet mix to dry ingredients in the bowl, and stir gently until well combined.

7. Spoon mix into muffin tray. Place in the oven and bake for 20–30 minutes, or until you stick a skewer in and it comes out clean.

8. Remove from oven and let muffins sit in the tray for a few minutes, before removing and placing on a cooling rack.

Note: If you are using rice bran or macadamia oil, add with the honey and rice milk, not at the start.

Labna

Labna is a cheese which is easily made from yoghurt. It has the benefits of containing good bacteria that is beneficial for your gut, and is easier to digest than most other cheeses.

What you'll need
Muslin cloth for hanging

Pot or bowl to catch liquid

Ingredients
Plain probiotic, full-fat organic yoghurt

Optional
You can mix in pepper, herbs, chilli, garlic, or anything else you might like into the yoghurt to make a flavoured labna

Method
1. Place the amount of yoghurt that you wish to make into cheese onto the muslin, then bunch the ends and hang with a bowl beneath it to catch the water (a pot with a lid can work well for this).
2. Leave overnight, or until the cheese has become firm and most of the liquid has been drained. (If you live in a warmer climate, you may need to hang it in the fridge.)
3. Store in a sterile, airtight container in the fridge.

Serving suggestions
- Rolled into small balls and tossed through a salad with baby spinach, roast pumpkin, capsicum and olive oil
- On a rye or brown rice cracker of your choice with smoked salmon and cracked pepper
- As a dip mixed with avocado, paprika, garlic and lemon juice served with carrot and celery sticks

Exercise resources

Exercise types

Exercise	Type	Pros	Cons
Brisk walking	Moderate aerobic	Can be done anywhere Can be done ad-hoc Good for general fitness Easy to fit in to routine Weight-bearing Strengthens legs	Not the best for weight loss Doesn't get heart rate up very high May be too low intensity (unless hilly)
Swimming	Moderate aerobic	Easy on body Good for those with injuries or joint pain Cardiovascular fitness Uses whole body Helps you focus on breathing	Regular swimming in public pools increases chlorine exposure (see page 88) Not weight-bearing
Cycling	Moderate to vigorous aerobic	Cardiovascular fitness Strengthens legs Strengthens core (if riding outside) Weight-bearing but gentle on joints	Can cause hip problems and back pain without proper care Riding in traffic may increase toxin exposure

Exercise	Type	Pros	Cons
Cycling	Moderate to vigorous aerobic	Can be your means of transport – combining exercise and travel	Can cause hip problems and back pain without proper care Riding in traffic may increase toxin exposure
Mowing the lawn	Moderate aerobic	Chores and exercise done at the same time! Exercises top and bottom half of the body	Noise can affect hearing – wear protective earplugs
Running/ jogging	Vigorous aerobic	Cardiovascular fitness Easy to track fitness level Can join events/races for motivation Weight-bearing	Hard on knees and ankles Can lead to tightness or injury if don't stretch
Dancing	Moderate to vigorous	Fun way to get fit Helps to nurture your creative side You can use your whole body Helps with balance and coordination Cardiovascular fitness You can do it around your house!	Can be challenging to get started if you have to remember steps

Exercise	Type	Pros	Cons
Aerobics classes – Step/Body attack, etc.	Vigorous aerobic	Cardiovascular fitness Strengthens legs Weight-bearing Helps with coordination	Often not enough stretching afterwards – consider doing some extra Hard on knees and ankle joints Need a certain amount of coordination to get started
Free weights	Strengthening	Helps to improve muscle mass Great for weight loss Easy to incorporate at the end of other exercises	Need to learn technique or you can injure yourself Need to balance with stretching to avoid tightness
Strength work – Push ups, sit ups, squats, lunges, etc.	Strengthening	Easy to do – no special equipment required Helps to build muscle Can get heart rate up Weight-bearing (standing exercises)	Need to learn technique to avoid injury

Exercise	Type	Pros	Cons
Yoga	Strengthening and stretching	Benefits nearly everyone Relaxing Helps to improve flexibility Teaches you how to breathe properly Helps to tone the body Weight bearing Strengthens core	Can be tough if you're very stiff Some people find it too slow moving – try dynamic (fast moving) yoga if this is you
Pilates	Strengthening	Best core strengthener Helps to tone body Helps to improve breathing Strengthens pelvic floor	Not weight bearing May be boring if you prefer a faster pace
Team sports – Football, netball, soccer, volleyball, etc.	Moderate to vigorous aerobic	Fun way to get fit Team schedule means you won't miss your exercise Good for building friendships and social circle	If not experienced may need some training Injury is more likely, especially in contact sports

Exercise	Type	Pros	Cons
Team sports – Football, netball, soccer, volleyball, etc.	Moderate to vigorous aerobic	Short bursts of intensity are good for your heart Cardiovascular fitness If strategic it will work your mind too	If not experienced may need some training Injury is more likely, especially in contact sports
Boxercise (as opposed to boxing, which is not recommended for healthy exercise due to risk of injury)	Moderate to vigorous aerobic and strengthening	Cardiovascular fitness Improves coordination Upper and lower body strengthening	Need to have special gloves Can put strain on wrists
Surfing	Moderate aerobic	Cardiovascular fitness Shoulder and back strength Core strengthening The ocean is cleansing and you'll absorb minerals from the water	You need to live near the beach Equipment can be costly Weather and surf conditions may prevent you from going out You may take a while to learn the skill

Exercise	Type	Pros	Cons
Kayaking/ rowing	Moderate aerobic	Can be done as a leisure activity Strengthens upper body Cardiovascular fitness	Need equipment and to be by water to do it Need to use the right technique to avoid back pain
Golf	Moderate aerobic	Lots of walking helps with cardiovascular fitness Strengthens upper body, legs and abdomen May help with stress release	Can be expensive Need to learn the skill Back pain is common

Exercise plans

Exercise plan 1 – building up slowly

Week one
Every morning before work, or every afternoon after work, go for a ten-minute walk. Do some gentle stretching afterwards. Try to do on the weekend as well as during the week.

Week two
Increase to a fifteen-minute walk, increasing your speed every day. Stretch afterwards, trying to hold the stretches for longer

Week three
Increase to twenty minutes a day. Try to include hills or some light jogging to get your heart rate up at least once. Stretch out afterwards.

Week four
Aim to do thirty minutes of brisk walking at least four times per week. Work your way up to include some jogging or hills. Continue to stretch out afterwards.

Exercise plan 2 – More intensive
This plan involves the use of a personal trainer or gym classes. If you are well-versed in this type of exercise you could make your own routine (or get your PT to set you up with one and do it yourself).

Week one
- One PT session, yoga or gym class, *and*
- One thirty-minute session at home involving cardio

(walking, jogging, cycling, treadmill, cross trainer) and
weights (free weights, push ups, sit ups, squats).

Week two
- Two PT sessions, yoga or gym classes, *and*
- One thirty-minute session at home.

Week three
- Three PT, yoga, or gym sessions.

ABOUT KATHERINE MASLEN

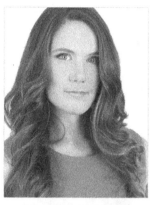

Katherine Maslen is a naturopath and nutritionist on a mission to empower others to live a better life through great health. After obtaining a dual bachelor degree in naturopathy and herbal medicine, Katherine has been spent over nine years helping people achieve amazing health from naturopathic care. She is passionate about giving her patients usable real-life tools to help them feel good again so they can live life the way that they want to.

Katherine has personally helped over 2,500 people with all kinds of health complaints – from fatigue and minor digestive discomfort to infertility and chronic autoimmune disease. Through Katherine's wide range of clients she has developed an in-depth understanding of the human body and what it takes to correct disease.

Katherine is also the principal and founder of the integrated health clinic Brisbane Natural Health (www.brisbanenaturalhealth. com.au), where she and her team help hundreds of patients every week to get well with their innovative approach to wellness.

Katherine is a public advocate of natural health and has presented to many organisations on health topics. She has appeared on the Channel 9 Today show, multiple radio outlets and is frequently interviewed for articles in publications like Wellbeing Magazine, Good Health Magazine, Marie Claire and Australian newspapers.

A mother, wife, business owner, private practitioner and author, Katherine knows what it is like to have to juggle a busy life while still maintaining your health. Katherine is known for inspiring others to improve their health in a practical, easy-to-understand way.

Katherine is available for TV, radio and print media opportunities and speaking engagements. Learn more about Katherine at www.katherinemaslen.com.

Want more of Katherine? You can get some through these channels...

1. Visit her website www.katherinemaslen.com and join the email list for regular health inspiration straight to your inbox.
2. Subscribe to Katherine's YouTube channel, *2 Minutes to Health* where you'll learn something new each week to further your health. Katherine talks about specific foods, diet tips, lifestyle advice and current health topics. Go to youtube.com/2MinutesToHealth to subscribe.
3. Follow Katherine on social media. Either go to www.katherinemaslen.com/getsocial for links, or follow...
   - Facebook – facebook.com/KatherineMaslenNaturopath
   - Twitter – @katherinemaslen
   - Instagram – @katherinemaslen
   - Google Plus – Katherine Maslen – Naturopath and Herbalist
4. Get a one-on-one consultation with Katherine or one of her hand-picked team members at Brisbane Natural Health, in person or via Skype. Go to www.brisbanenaturalhealth.com.au

CPSIA information can be obtained
at www.ICGtesting.com
Printed in the USA
LVHW111558260521
688573LV00005B/54